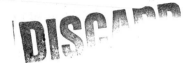

Physical Therapist Assistant

BOARD REVIEW

Brad Fortinberry, PT
Director of Sports Medicine
Southwest Center for Rehabilitation
Southwest Mississippi Regional Medical Center
McComb, Mississippi

Michael Dunaway, PT
Staff Physical Therapist
Southwest Center for Rehabilitation
Southwest Mississippi Regional Medical Center
McComb, Mississippi

Justin Boyd, LPTA
Staff Physical Therapist Assistant
Gilbert's Home Health
McComb, Mississippi

HANLEY & BELFUS, INC.
An Affiliate of Elsevier

HANLEY & BELFUS, INC.
An Affiliate of Elsevier

The Curtis Center
Independence Square West
Philadelphia, Pennsylvania 19106

Note to the reader: Although the information in this book has been carefully reviewed for correctness of dosage and indications, neither the authors nor the publisher can accept any legal responsibility for any errors or omissions that may be made. Neither the publisher nor authors make any warranty, expressed or implied, with respect to the material contained herein. Before prescribing any drug, the reader must review the manufacturer's current product information (package inserts) for accepted indications, absolute dosage recommendations, and other information pertinent to the safe and effective use of the product described. This is especially important when drugs are given in combination or as an adjunct to other forms of therapy.

Library of Congress Control Number: 2003110160

PHYSICAL THERAPIST ASSISTANT BOARD REVIEW   ISBN 1-56053-605-5

Printed in the United States

Last digit is the print number: 9 8 7 6 5 4 3 2 1

Contents

Preface

When reviewing material for the National Physical Therapist Assistant Exam (NPTAE), we were disappointed by the lack of appropriate study manuals. The manuals available often contained many errors or contained questions that were not the type of functional questions that appeared on the actual exam. This motivated us to create the *Physical Therapist Assistant Board Review,* which contains 400 well-researched questions, answers, and explanations that we feel more closely resemble the style of questions on the NPTAE.

In preparation for the NPTAE, the reader should remember that most of the questions will be in "scenario" format. There are very few, if any, questions such as, "What nerve innervates the rectus femoris?" The question would more likely be, "Which motions at the knee would be limited if there was an injury at the L2–L4 level?" Although the student must know the correct nerve and muscle combination to answer correctly, the question is presented in a more "real world" format.

A bibliography of the resources used in preparing this review manual is located at the end of the book.

It is our hope that you will find the *Physical Therapist Assistant Board Review* a valuable resource when preparing for the NPTAE.

Brad Fortinberry, PT
Michael Dunaway, PT
Justin Boyd, PTA

EXAM
QUESTIONS

Question 1.

A patient with dysarthria and dysphagia is being treated by physical and speech therapy services. The physical therapist assistant (PTA) can aid the patient in which of the following ways?

A. Provide posture control exercises, teach the patient swallowing techniques of thin liquids, provide facial musculature exercises, and provide good verbal interaction.
B. Teach the patient to have good eye contact, provide facial musculature exercises, and teach increased head and trunk control.
C. Provide posture control exercises, provide multiple sources of stimuli during exercise sessions, teach the patient swallowing techniques of thin liquids, and teach the patient swallowing techniques for prescribed medications in capsular form.
D. None of the above

Question 2.

A PTA is aiding a patient with an injury at the C5 level in performing an effective cough. The patient has experienced significant neurological damage and is unable to perform an independent, effective cough. If the patient is in a supine position, which of the following methods is most likely to produce an effective cough?

A. The PTA places the heel of one hand just above the xiphoid process, instructs the patient to take a deep breath while pressing down moderately on the sternum, and instructs the patient to cough.
B. The PTA places the heel of one hand, reinforced with the other hand, just above the xiphoid process; instructs the patient to take a deep breath; instructs the patient to hold the breath; and presses moderately as the patient coughs.
C. The PTA places the heel of one hand on the area just above the umbilicus, instructs the patient to take a deep breath, applies moderate pressure, and releases pressure just before the patient attempts to cough.
D. The PTA places the heel of one hand just above the umbilicus, instructs the patient to take a deep breath, and applies moderate pressure while instructing the patient to cough.

Question 3.

A physical therapist has asked an assistant to treat a 57-year-old woman with a diagnosis of spondylolisthesis who is complaining of low back pain. The plan of care initiated by the therapist includes TENS (transcutaneous neuromuscular stimulation) application with two electrodes lateral to the spinal cord on each side of the area of pain, education on body mechanics during functional activities, and instruction to the patient on performing a home exercise program focusing on flexion exercises. Which of the following is the correct course of action of the PTA after reviewing the plan of care?

A. Perform the tasks as outlined in the plan of care.
B. Perform all tasks with the exception of the TENS application (before consulting with the physical therapist) because it is contraindicated.
C. Perform all tasks as outlined but suggest to the physical therapist that the home program should focus on extension exercises.
D. Consult with the physical therapist because two of the three tasks listed are contraindicated for this patient.

Question 4.

A PTA is treating a patient with an injury at the T8 level and compromised function of the diaphragm. If no abdominal binder is available, what is the most likely position of comfort to allow the patient to breathe most efficiently?

A. Sitting position
B. Semi-Fowler's position
C. Upright standing position using a tilt table
D. Supine

Question 5.

A PTA is using electrical stimulation to increase a patient's quadriceps strength, as suggested by the supervising physical therapist. Which of the following is the best protocol?

A. Electrodes placed over the superior/lateral quadriceps and the vastus medialis obliquus—stimulation on for 15 seconds and then off for 15 seconds
B. Electrodes over the femoral nerve in the proximal quadriceps and the vastus medialis obliquus—stimulation on for 50 seconds and then off for 10 seconds
C. Electrodes over the vastus medialis obliquus and superior/lateral quadriceps—stimulation frequency set between 50–80 Hz (pps)
D. Electrodes over the femoral nerve in the proximal quadriceps and the vastus medialis obliquus—stimulation frequency set between 50–80 Hz (pps)

Question 6.

A therapist is applying biofeedback electrodes to the quadriceps of a stroke patient's lower extremity. The intention of the therapist is to strengthen the quadriceps in an effort to improve knee stability during ambulation. The therapist is also explaining to the patient's family what is actually taking place in the nervous system when using this method. Which of the following is correct information to convey to this family?

A. Visual input is being sent to the central nervous system (CNS) via efferent nerves. Motor input is being sent from the CNS via afferent nerves to the muscle.
B. Visual input is being sent to the CNS via afferent nerves. Motor input is being sent from the CNS via efferent nerves to the muscle.
C. Visual input is being sent to the peripheral nervous system (PNS) via efferent nerves. Motor input is being sent from the CNS via afferent nerves to the muscle.
D. Visual input is being sent to the PNS via afferent nerves. Motor input is being sent from the PNS via efferent nerves to the muscle.

Question 7.

A PTA is assessing a patient's strength in the right shoulder. The patient has 0° of active shoulder abduction in the standing position. In the supine position, the patient has 42° of active shoulder abduction and 175° of pain-free passive shoulder abduction. What is the correct manual muscle testing grade for the patient's shoulder abduction?

A. 3−/5 (fair−)
B. 2+/5 (poor+)
C. 2−/5 (poor−)
D. 1/5 (trace)

Question 8.

A patient has traumatically dislocated the tibia directly posteriorly during an automobile accident. Which of the following structures is the least likely to be injured?

A. Tibial nerve
B. Popliteal artery
C. Common peroneal nerve
D. Anterior cruciate ligament

Question 9.

A PTA is treating a patient who recently received a below-knee amputation. The assistant notices in the patient's chart that a psychiatrist has stated that the patient is in the second stage of the grieving process. Which stage of the grieving process is this patient most likely exhibiting?

A. Denial
B. Acceptance
C. Depression
D. Anger

Question 10.

A PTA is asked by a physical therapist to treat a patient with congestive heart failure in an outpatient cardiac rehabilitation facility. Which of the following signs and symptoms should the assistant not expect?

A. Stenosis of the mitral valve
B. Orthopnea
C. Decreased preload of the right heart
D. Pulmonary edema

Question 11.

A patient is scheduled to receive passive range of motion (ROM) to the extremities. This patient is in the intensive care unit of the hospital as a result of a blunt force injury to the head. When reviewing the chart, the therapist discovers that at the time of arrival to the hospital, bleeding occurred between the outer layer of membrane, covering the brain, and the middle layer of membrane. This type of hematoma is commonly referred to as a/an _____ hematoma. The outer membrane is called the _____, and the middle layer is called the _____.

A. Subarachnoid, arachnoid membrane, dura mater
B. Subdural, dura mater, arachnoid membrane
C. Epidural, pia mater, arachnoid membrane
D. Epidural, dura mater, pia mater

Question 12.

A PTA is attempting to gain external rotation ROM in a patient's right shoulder. The assistant decides to use contract–relax–contract antagonist. In what order should the following rotator cuff muscles contract to successfully perform this movement?

A. Infraspinatus—teres minor
B. Subscapularis—supraspinatus
C. Teres minor—infraspinatus
D. Supraspinatus—subscapularis

Question 13.

A PTA is instructing a student in writing a SOAP note. The student has misplaced the following phrase: "Patient reports a functional goal of returning to playing baseball in 5 weeks." Where should this phrase be placed in a SOAP note?

A. Subjective
B. Objective
C. Assessment
D. Plan

Question 14.

A PTA is treating a patient who received an above-elbow amputation 2 years ago. The prosthesis has a split cable that controls the elbow and the terminal device. With this type of prosthesis, the patient must first lock the elbow to allow the cable to activate the terminal device. This is accomplished with what movements?

A. Extending the humerus and elevating the scapula
B. Extending the humerus and retracting the scapula
C. Extending the humerus and protracting the scapula
D. Extending the humerus and depressing the scapula

Question 15.

A PTA is scheduled to treat a patient with cerebral palsy who has been classified as a spastic quadriplegic. What type of orthopedic deformity should the therapist expect to see in the patient's feet?

A. Talipes equinovalgus
B. Talipes equinovarus *(club foot)*
C. Clubfeet
D. B and C

Question 16.

A PTA assistant is giving a pulmonary patient instructions on energy conservation when he notices that the patient is not breathing normally. The patient is quickly instructed to use the pursed-lip breathing technique to slow down his rapid breathing rate. The rapid rate of breathing is referred to as tachypnea, and normal rate of breathing is referred to as _____.

A. Apnea
B. Eupnea
C. Apneusis
D. Orthopnea

Question 17.

A PTA is instructing a patient in the use of a wrist-driven prehension orthotic device. What must be done to achieve opening of the involved hand?

A. Actively extend the wrist
B. Passively extend the wrist
C. Actively flex the wrist
D. Passively flex the wrist

Question 18.

Which of the following is the most appropriate orthotic device for a patient with excessive foot pronation during static standing?

A. Scaphoid pad
B. Metatarsal pad
C. Metatarsal bar
D. Rocker bar

Question 19.

A PTA is teaching a patient ROM exercise for the knee joint. The patient suffered an injury 6 months earlier, which consisted of the patella tendon pulling off a portion of the tibial tuberosity. This is described as what type of fracture?

A. Greenstick
B. Comminuted
C. Complicated
D. Avulsion

Question 20.

After arriving at the home of a home health patient, a primary nurse informs the PTA that she has activated emergency medical services. The nurse found the patient in what appears to be a diabetic coma. Which of the following is most likely not one of the patient's signs?

A. Skin flush
B. Rapid pulse
C. Weak pulse
D. High blood pressure

Question 21.

A PTA is treating a patient who is having gait difficulty. The patient received a total hip replacement 1 year ago and still has an obvious limp. The gait pattern demonstrated by the patient consists of a drop of the pelvis on the uninvolved side during the stance phase of the involved lower extremity. The patient also has a lateral trunk lean toward the involved side during single limb support on the involved lower extremity. The physical therapist has chosen an appropriate treatment plan for this patient that involves strengthening of the bilateral lower extremities, with an emphasis on the _____ muscle on the _____ side, which is the muscle most responsible for this patient's gait deviation.

A. Gluteus medius, involved
B. Gluteus medius, uninvolved
C. Gluteus maximus, involved
D. Gluteus maximus, uninvolved

Question 22.

A PTA is treating a patient who has a diagnosis of right shoulder adhesive capsulitis. This patient has painful end-feels in all planes in the involved shoulder. The physical therapist initiated a plan of care consisting of ROM pulley exercises, grade IV inferior glide joint mobilization, rotator cuff resistive theraband exercises, and establishment of a home exercise program. Which of the above is the most important for this patient?

A. ROM pulley exercises
B. Grade IV inferior glide joint mobilization
C. Rotator cuff resistive theraband exercises
D. Establishment of a home exercise program

Question 23.

Which of the following articulates with the second cuneiform?

A. Navicular
B. Talus
C. First metatarsal
D. Cuboid

Question 24.

Which of the following is the most vulnerable position for dislocation of the hip?

A. 30° hip extension, 30° hip adduction, and minimal internal rotation
B. 30° hip flexion, 30° hip adduction, and minimal external rotation
C. 30° hip flexion, 30° hip abduction, and minimal external rotation
D. 30° hip extension, 30° hip abduction, and minimal external rotation

Question 25.

Observing a patient in a standing position, a PTA notes that an angulation deformity of the right knee causes it to be located medially in relation to the left hip and left foot. This condition is commonly referred to as:

A. Genu varum
B. Genu valgum
C. Pes cavus
D. None of the above

Question 26.

A patient at an outpatient facility experiences the onset of a grand mal seizure. Which of the following is the most appropriate course of action by the PTA?

A. Assist the patient to a lying position, move away close furniture, loosen tight clothes, and prop the patient's mouth open.
B. Assist the patient to a lying position, move away close furniture, and loosen tight clothes.
C. Assist the patient to a seated position, move away close furniture, and loosen tight clothes.
D. Assist the patient to a seated position, move away close furniture, loosen tight clothing, and prop the patient's mouth open.

Question 27.

A PTA is beginning treatment on a patient diagnosed with right-side hemiplegia. The therapist notes that the patient is able to understand spoken language but is unable to speak well. Most of the patient's words are incomprehensible. The patient also has difficulty in naming simple objects. What type of aphasia does the patient most likely have?

A. Anomic aphasia
B. Broca's aphasia
C. Crossed aphasia
D. Wernicke's aphasia

Question 28.

Which of the following acts forced all federally supported facilities to increase corridor width to a minimum of 54 inches to accommodate wheelchairs?

A. Americans with Disabilities Act (ADA)
B. National Healthcare and Resource Development Act
C. Civil Rights Act
D. Older Americans Act (title III)

Question 29.

A 17-year-old boy has received an anterior cruciate ligament reconstruction 2 weeks ago. He is now scheduled to begin outpatient rehabilitation. The PTA, aware that the patient is being admitted tomorrow, can anticipate from the above information only that this patient will most likely begin with the following list of exercises with the exception of which one?

A. Patella mobilization
B. Passive knee extension
C. Terminal knee extensions
D. Isometric quadriceps contractions

Question 30.

A PTA is treating the ankle of a 15-year-old athlete. The patient has suffered a sprain in a track event the night before. The PTA has received a request from the supervising therapist to apply compression wrapping to the involved ankle and foot, elevate the involved foot above the heart with the patient in the supine position, and apply ice for approximately 10 minutes. Just before carrying out the treatment, the therapist assistant notices that the ankle is swollen, red in color, and warm to the touch. Which of the following would be the correct course of action for the therapist assistant?

A. Ask the supervising therapist to reassess the ankle before treating.
B. Ask the supervising therapist if the compression wrapping can be omitted from the treatment.
C. Perform the treatment as planned.
D. Consult with the supervising therapist because the supine positioning is contraindicated.

Question 31.

A PTA is assessing radial deviation ROM at the wrist. The correct position of the goniometer should be the proximal arm aligned with the forearm and the distal arm aligned with the third metacarpal. What should be used as the axis point?

A. Lunate
B. Scaphoid
C. Capitate
D. Triquetrum

Question 32.

Which of the following tissues absorbs the least amount of an ultrasound beam at 1 MHz?

A. Bone
B. Skin
C. Muscle
D. Blood

Question 33.

A PTA is treating a home health patient for the third time in 1 week. The patient has been performing lower extremity strengthening exercises in a standing position with the support of the PTA and a standard walker. The patient's program, in addition to gait training, has consisted of active hip flexion, active hip extension, active hip abduction, mini squats, and active plantar flexion (toe raises). The patient is complaining, however, of increased "soreness" in the calf region of bilateral lower extremities. The patient's calf is not unusually warm to the touch, but he does complain of severe pain with active dorsiflexion in bilateral calves. Which of the following would be the best course of action for the PTA?

A. Only perform stretching exercises to the calf and ankle pumps.
B. Call the supervising therapist before continuing treatment.
C. Continue as normal with the patient's original program.
D. Perform supine lower extremity exercises and do not provide gait training this session.

Question 34.

A 27-year-old woman is referred to a physical therapy clinic with a diagnosis of torticollis. The right sternocleidomastoid is involved. What is the most likely position of the patient's cervical spine?

A. Right lateral cervical flexion and left cervical rotation
B. Right cervical rotation and right lateral cervical flexion
C. Left cervical rotation and left lateral cervical flexion
D. Left lateral cervical flexion and right cervical rotation

Question 35.

A PTA is providing passive ROM to a patient's right elbow in an effort to gain full passive extension. The patient has a long history of rheumatoid arthritis and currently lacks 12 degrees of passive elbow extension on the involved side. The therapist assistant notices a bone-to-bone end-feel when performing passive ROM into elbow extension. The therapist also notices that the uninvolved elbow lacks 6° of full passive elbow extension. The patient is unable to reliably provide a subjective history, and no family members are currently present. Which of the following is the best course of action for this PTA?

A. The PTA should consult with the supervising therapist about beginning passive ROM on the uninvolved elbow as well.
B. The PTA should consult with the supervising therapist about discontinuing efforts to increase elbow extension passively on the involved side.
C. The intensity of passive ROM should be increased on the involved side until bilateral elbow extension is equal.
D. The current treatment plan on the involved elbow should be continued.

Question 36.

When reviewing a patient's chart, a PTA determines that the patient has a condition in which the cauda equina is in a fluid-filled sac protruding from the back. What form of spina bifida does the patient most likely have?

A. Meningocele
B. Meningomyelocele
C. Spina bifida occulta
D. None of the above

Question 37.

A physical therapist instructs a PTA to teach a patient how to ascend and descend the front steps of her home. After first exercising the patient at her home, the assistant realizes that, because of the patient's increased size and severe dynamic balance deficits, training on the steps is unsafe at this time. The assistant contacts the therapist by telephone, and the physical therapist instructs the assistant to continue with ambulation. Which of the following is the best course of action by the assistant?

A. The assistant should cautiously attempt step training.
B. The assistant should recruit the family members to assist with step training.
C. The assistant should discontinue step training until he or she and the supervising therapist can both be present.
D. The assistant should contact the physician and seek further instructions.

Question 38.

A physician instructs a PTA to educate a patient about the risk factors of atherosclerosis.
Which of the following is the most inappropriate list?

A. Diabetes, male gender, and excessive alcohol
B. Genetic predisposition, smoking, and sedentary lifestyle
C. Stress and inadequate exercise
D. Obesity, smoking, and hypotension

Question 39.

A diabetic patient is exercising vigorously in an outpatient clinic. The patient informs a PTA
that he received insulin immediately before the exercise session. If the patient goes into a
hypoglycemic coma, which of the following is not a likely sign?

A. Pallor
B. Shallow respirations
C. Bounding pulse
D. Dry skin

Question 40.

A physician prescribes isotonic exercises for the left biceps brachii. Which of the following
exercises is in compliance with this order?

A. Biceps curls with the patient actively and independently using a 5-pound dumbbell as
   resistance
B. Rhythmic stabilization for the left elbow
C. Elbow flexion at 90° per second with speed controlled by a work simulator
D. None of the above

Question 41.

While observing a patient who has just received a new left below-knee prosthesis, a PTA
notes that the toe of the prosthesis stays off the floor after heel strike. Which of the following
is an unlikely cause of this deviation?

A. The prosthetic foot is set too far anterior.
B. The prosthetic foot is set in too much dorsiflexion.
C. The heel wedge is too stiff.
D. The prosthetic foot is outset too much.

Question 42.

A patient asks a PTA whether she should be concerned that her 4-month-old infant cannot roll from his back to his stomach. The most appropriate response to the parent is:

A. "This is probably nothing to be concerned about because, although it varies, infants can usually perform this task by 10 months of age."
B. "This is probably nothing to be concerned about because, although it varies, infants can usually perform this task by 5 months of age."
C. "Your infant probably needs further evaluation by a specialist because, although it varies, infants can usually perform this task at 2 months of age."
D. "Your infant probably needs further evaluation by a specialist because, although it varies, infants can usually perform this task at birth."

Question 43.

A PTA is working with a patient that has a diagnosis of Guillain-Barré syndrome. The patient is just starting therapy at this particular rehabilitation facility and has already received approximately 4 months of therapy at other facilities. From this information only, which of the following is most likely correct?

A. This patient has a poor prognosis and will likely decline significantly over the next 2 months.
B. This patient will likely improve over the next couple months to the point of full or almost complete recovery.
C. This patient will likely live no more than 7 years, with a slow, steady decrease in mobility.
D. This patient has a good prognosis, but continued therapy is a contraindication for this patient.

Question 44.

During the treatment of an infant, a PTA observes that with passive flexion of the head the infant actively flexes the arms and actively extends the legs. Which of the following reflexes is being observed?

A. Protective extension
B. Optical righting
C. Symmetrical tonic neck
D. Labyrinthine head righting

Question 45.

A PTA has just discovered that, because of poor positioning of a 62-year-old man during a rotator cuff repair, the patient suffered damage to the common peroneal nerve. This information alone should clue the assistant that the patient will probably exhibit which of the following?

A. Circumduction during ambulation
B. Increased internal rotation of the involved shoulder with the forearm pronated and the wrist and hand fixed in a flexed position
C. Loss of full shoulder external rotation on the involved side even after extensive rehabilitation
D. Trendelenburg gait

Question 46.

During a case conference, a respiratory therapist indicates that the patient has a low expiratory reserve volume. What does this mean?

A. The volume of air remaining in the lungs after a full expiration is low.
B. The volume of air in a breath during normal breathing is low.
C. The volume of air forcefully expired after a forceful inspiration is low.
D. The amount of air expired after a resting expiration is low.

Question 47.

A PTA is reviewing the written evaluation of a patient who has suffered a recent knee injury. The assistant notices that the structure damaged prevents excessive anterior displacement of the tibia on the femur. Knowing this, the therapist would expect all of the following tests, with the exception of which, to show positive results?

A. Anterior drawer
B. Lachman's
C. Pivot shift
D. McMurray

Question 48.

A patient is positioned in the supine position. The involved left upper extremity is positioned by the PTA in 90° of shoulder flexion. The assistant applies resistance into shoulder flexion and then extension. No movement takes place. The assistant instructs the patient to "hold" when resistance is applied in both directions. Which of the following proprioceptive neuromuscular facilitation techniques is being used?

A. Repeated contractions
B. Hold-relax
C. Rhythmic stabilization
D. Contract-relax

Question 49.

A PTA is observing the evaluation being performed by a physical therapist on a patient who has a fractured vertebral body. The therapist is palpating the spinal musculature at the level of the spine of the scapula. The patient indicates that this is the area of increased pain and is the approximate level of the fractured vertebrae. Which vertebra is at this level?

A. T2
B. T3
C. T7
D. None of the above

Question 50.

An infant with Erb's palsy presents with the involved upper extremity in which of the following positions?

A. Hand supinated and wrist extended
B. Hand supinated and wrist flexed
C. Hand pronated and wrist extended
D. Hand pronated and wrist flexed

Question 51.

A patient presents to therapy with a deformity of the right hand. The involved finger is in the position of extension at the proximal interphalangeal joint and flexion at the distal interphalangeal joint. Which of the following is the correct term that describes this type of deformity?

A. Claw hand
B. Swan neck
C. Boutonnière
D. Dupuytren's

Question 52.

The physical therapist is performing an orthopedic test that involves (1) placing the patient in a sidelying position, (2) placing the superior lower extremity in hip extension and hip abduction, (3) placing the knee of the superior lower extremity in 90° of flexion, and (4) allowing the superior lower extremity to drop into adduction. Failure of the superior lower extremity to drop indicates a tight:

A. Iliopsoas
B. Rectus femoris
C. Iliotibial band
D. Hamstring

Question 53.

A PTA is scheduled to instruct a diabetic patient in performing a home exercise program. The assistant is informed, at the beginning of her conversation with the physical therapist, that this patient has been controlling diabetes with diet. Before the conversation continues, the assistant knows:

A. This patient is probably a type I diabetic.
B. This patient is probably a type II diabetic.
C. This patient may be either a type I or type II diabetic.
D. There is not enough information to make any conclusions.

Question 54.

A physical therapist has informed a PTA that it will be necessary to use a platform walker when gait training their next scheduled patient. The assistant knows from this information that:

A. The patient is short in height.
B. The patient has severe balance deficits.
C. The patient has some problem with an upper extremity that has limited weight-bearing ability on that extremity or has limited the functional mobility of that upper extremity.
D. This patient fatigues easily and needs a walker that has a built-in seat.

Question 55.

A PTA is gait training a patient and notes that the pelvis drops inferiorly on the right during the mid-swing phase of the right lower extremity. The patient also leans laterally to the left with the upper trunk during this phase. Which of the following is the most likely cause of this deviation?

A. Weak right gluteus medius
B. Weak right adductor longus
C. Weak left gluteus medius
D. Weak left adductor longus

Question 56.

A PTA is attempting to convey information to an observing student regarding writing and signing discharge summaries. Which of the following statements is true?

A. A physical therapist must sign a discharge summary after the assistant when the summary is written by an assistant.
B. A physical therapist assistant cannot legally write a discharge summary.
C. A PTA does not need the signature of a supervising therapist on a discharge summary written by the assistant.
D. The physical therapist must sign first, then the assistant, when the discharge summary is written by the assistant.

Question 57.

The PTA observes a patient with the later stages of Parkinson's disease during ambulation. Which of the following characteristics is the assistant most likely observing?

A. Shuffling gait
B. Increased step width
C. Difficulty initiating the first steps
D. A and C

Question 58.

A PTA is treating a patient who has suffered a traumatic brain injury. The therapist is using a treatment technique that consists of tracing different letters and numbers on the patient's hand. There is also a shield present, preventing the patient from actually seeing the letters and numbers as they are being traced. This technique will improve:

A. Barognosis
B. Stereognosis
C. Texture recognition
D. Graphesthesia

Question 59.

A physical therapy technician calls a PTA immediately to the other side of the outpatient clinic. The physical therapy assistant discovers a 37-year-old woman lying face down on the floor. Which of the following sequence of events is most appropriate for this situation?

A. Have someone call 911, determine unresponsiveness, establish an airway, and assess breathing (look/listen/feel)
B. Determine unresponsiveness, have someone call 911, establish an airway, and assess breathing (look/listen/feel)
C. Have someone call 911, determine unresponsiveness, assess breathing (look/listen/feel), and establish an airway
D. Determine unresponsiveness, have someone call 911, assess breathing (look/listen/feel), and establish an airway

Question 60.

A patient is referred to physical therapy services for care of a burn wound on the left foot. The majority of the wound is anesthetic. There is significant eschar formation over the dorsum of the involved foot, and moderate subcutaneous tissue damage is present. What is the most likely classification of this burn?

A. Electrical
B. Superficial partial thickness
C. Deep partial thickness
D. Full thickness

Question 61.

A patient is sitting over the edge of a table and performing active knee extension exercises using an ankle weight as resistance. This exercise demonstrates what class lever?

A. First class
B. Second class
C. Third class
D. Fourth class

Question 62.

A PTA is treating a patient who has a diagnosis of Dupuytren's contracture. The plan of care currently consists of passive ROM provided the therapist, fluidotherapy, and a home exercise program consisting of stretching exercises. This program should initially focus on achieving:

A. Passive extension of the elbow
B. Active supination of the forearm
C. Passive extension of the wrist
D. None of the above

Question 63.

A PTA is asked to estimate the percentage of a patient's body that has been burned. The patient is a 32-year-old man of normal size. Burns are located along the entire anterior surface of the face. The patient also burned the entire anterior portion of the right upper extremity in an attempt to guard himself from flames. Using the rule of nines, what percentage of the patient's body is burned?

A. 9%
B. 18%
C. 4.5%
D. 27%

Question 64.

A patient who has suffered a recent fracture of the right tibia and fibula has developed foot drop of the right foot during gait. Which nerve is causing this loss of motor function?

A. Posterior tibial
B. Superficial peroneal
C. Deep peroneal
D. Anterior tibial

Question 65.

A PTA is treating a patient who has dysfunction of the right upper extremity. The patient has a diagnosis of reflex sympathetic dystrophy and presents with the following signs and symptoms: decreased hypersensitivity, normal temperature, marked muscle atrophy, and smooth skin. The patient is in what stage of reflex sympathetic dystrophy?

A. Acute
B. Dystrophic
C. Atrophic
D. None of the above

Question 66.

A PTA begins treatment for a 72-year-old woman who has suffered a recent stroke. The physical therapist has determined that this patient needs to focus on pre-gait activities. Which of the proprioceptive neuromuscular facilitation (PNF) diagonals best encourages normal gait?

A. D1
B. D2
C. PNF is contraindicated
D. Pelvic PNF patterns only

Question 67.

A patient is scheduled to undergo extremely risky heart surgery. The patient seems really worried. During the treatment session, the patient and family look to the PTA for comfort. Which of the following is an appropriate response from the therapist to the patient?

A. "Don't worry; everything will be okay."
B. "Your physician is the best, and he will take care of you."
C. "I know it must be upsetting to face such a difficult situation. Your family and friends are here to support you."
D. "Try not to worry. Worrying increases your blood pressure and heart rate, which are two factors that need to be stabilized before surgery."

Question 68.

A PTA is gait training a patient who has severe bruising of one of the quadricep muscles. The assistant notices that during ambulation, without an assistive device, the patient has an abnormally short distance between left heel strike and the successive left heel strike. Which quadricep is most likely bruised, and which of the following best describes the gait deviation in reference to the left lower extremity?

A. Left quadriceps; a decreased step duration
B. Left quadriceps; a decrease in single limb support time
C. Right quadriceps; a decreased step length
D. Right quadriceps; a decreased stride length

Question 69.

To facilitate development of a functional tenodesis grip in a patient with spinal cord injury, the treatment plan should include:

A. Stretching of the finger flexors and finger extensors
B. Stretching of the finger flexors
C. Allowing the finger flexors and finger extensors to shorten
D. Allowing the finger flexors to shorten

Question 70.

A PTA is performing a chart review and discovers that laboratory results reveal that the patient has malignant cancer. When treating the patient, the assistant is asked by the patient, "Did my lab results come back, and is the cancer malignant?" The appropriate response for the assistant is:

A. Tell the patient the truth and contact the social worker to assist in consultation of the family.
B. "It is inappropriate for me to comment on your diagnosis before the doctor has assessed the lab results and spoken to you first."
C. "The results are positive for malignant cancer, but I do not have the training to determine your prognosis."
D. Tell the patient the results are in, but therapist assistants are not allowed to speak on this matter.

Question 71.

A 16-year-old football player has returned from the physician with an order stating, "weight bearing as tolerated and wean off crutches." The patient received a left knee lateral meniscus repair 6 weeks earlier and has been non–weight bearing until receiving this last order. The assistant notices that with one crutch only, the patient has a significant limp. Which of the following would be the best set of instructions for this patient knowing the above information?

A. "Walk with one crutch on the right side until your next therapy session day after tomorrow."
B. "Start walking with one crutch on the right side approximately 1 hour beginning tomorrow and gradually increase the amount of time using one crutch versus two crutches each day."
C. "Walk with one crutch the rest of today and walk without crutches beginning tomorrow."
D. "Start placing more weight on the left leg, but walk as normally as possible using two crutches until your next session day after tomorrow."

Question 72.

The physical therapist is performing an orthopedic test on a 25-year-old man with the chief complaint of low back pain. The patient has positive Thomas test results. With this information, what might the assistant need to include in treatment?

A. Stretching of the hip abductors
B. Stretching of the hip adductors
C. Stretching of the hip extensors
D. Stretching of the hip flexors

Question 73.

A physician has contacted an outpatient facility to inquire about the status of one of her patients. The PTA has answered the call and is asked by the physician whether or not the patient is making adequate progress. Which of the following is the correct course of action by the PTA?

A. Have the physician hold until the physical therapist can answer his questions.
B. Inform the physician that a written progress report will be faxed to him immediately.
C. Answer the physician's question regarding the patient's progress.
D. Inform the physician that the physical therapist must inform him of the patient's progress, but he (the PTA) can tell the physician what type of exercises the patient has been performing.

Question 74.

A PTA is attempting to educate a patient on some of the signs and symptoms of rheumatoid arthritis. Which of the following would be incorrect information to convey to this patient?

A. Rheumatoid arthritis often causes more stiffness in the morning than in the evening.
B. Rheumatoid arthritis is a systemic condition.
C. Rheumatoid arthritis usually causes pain symmetrically.
D. Rheumatoid arthritis primarily affects the weight-bearing joints.

Question 75.

A 42-year-old construction worker received a burst fracture in the cervical spine when struck by a falling crossbeam. Proprioception is intact in bilateral lower extremities. The patient has bilateral loss of motor function and sensitivity to pain and temperature below the level of the lesion. This type of lesion is most typical of which of the following syndromes?

A. Central cord syndrome
B. Brown Sequard syndrome
C. Anterior cord syndrome
D. Conus medullaris syndrome

Question 76.

A PTA has just returned from a continuing education course offering new treatment techniques in wound care. The assistant would like to share the information with interested members of the hospital staff. What is the best way to share this information?

A. Prepare a handout on the new treatment techniques and give it to the members of the hospital staff.
B. Schedule a mandatory inservice during lunch for the entire hospital staff that participates in some form of wound care.
C. Post bulletins in view of all hospital staff and send memos to the department heads inviting everyone to attend an inservice during lunch.
D. Call each department head and invite him or her and their staff to an inservice during lunch.

Question 77.

A PTA is treating a patient in order to strengthen to the left knee quadriceps with isotonic exercises. Which of the following is not in this classification of exercise?

A. Terminal knee extensions
B. Wall sits
C. Mini squats
D. Stationary bike

Question 78.

In treatment of a 28-year-old pregnant woman, which of the following muscles should be the focus of the strengthening exercises to maintain a strong pelvic floor?

A. Piriformis, obturator internus, and pubococcygeus
B. Obturator internus, pubococcygeus, and coccygeus
C. Rectus abdominis, iliococcygeus, and piriformis
D. Iliococcygeus, pubococcygeus, and coccygeus

Question 79.

Which of the following is least likely in a woman in the eighth month of pregnancy?

A. Center of gravity anteriorly displaced
B. Heart rate decreased with rest and increased with activity (compared with heart rate before pregnancy)
C. Edema in bilateral lower extremities
D. Blood pressure increased by 5% (compared with blood pressure before pregnancy)

Question 80.

A physical therapist is evaluating a 36-year-old woman to fit her with the appropriate wheelchair. Recent injury caused C6 quadriplegia. A PTA is asked to assist the physical therapist in performing the measurements for this patient. What is the correct way to measure length of the footrests for the patient's permanent wheelchair?

A. From the patient's popliteal fossa to the heel and add 1 inch
B. From the patient's popliteal fossa to the heel and subtract 1 inch
C. From the patient's popliteal fossa to the first metatarsal head and add 1 inch
D. From the patient's popliteal fossa to the first metatarsal head and subtract 1 inch

Question 81.

A PTA is observing a patient performing biceps curls using a weight stack machine. The patient is able to perform 10 repetitions but appears to be fatiguing on the eleventh repetition. While performing the eleventh repetition, the patient is able to achieve full flexion. The patient then attempts to hold the machine at full elbow flexion but is unable, allowing the machine to slowly pull the elbow back into extension. What type of contraction is the patient performing when the machine is pulling the elbow into extension?

A. Isokinetic
B. Eccentric
C. Concentric
D. Isometric

Question 82.

A patient is suffering from rotator cuff impingement. The physical therapist has developed a plan of treatment that will emphasize strengthening of the muscles that help stabilize the humeral head in the glenoid fossa. Which of the follow muscles would contribute least in this task?

A. Infraspinatus
B. Teres minor
C. Middle deltoid
D. Subscapularis

Question 83.

A physician orders stage II cardiac rehabilitation for a patient. The orders are to exercise the patient below 7 metabolic equivalents (METs). Which of the following is a contraindicated activity?

A. Riding a stationary bike at approximately 5.5 mph
B. Descending a flight of stairs independently
C. Ironing
D. Ambulating independently at 5–6 mph

Question 84.

A patient has arrived for her appointment at an outpatient clinic. When first seen by the PTA, the patient is asked how she has been feeling since the last physical therapy session. The patient states, "I have really hurt in my calves since performing toes raises in the last session." The PTA includes this statement in the patient's SOAP note. In which section of the note should this statement be placed?

A. The S portion of the note because it is a statement from the patient
B. The O portion of the note because the patient has complained that part of the treatment session, toe raises, caused increased pain
C. The A portion of the note because the statement is an accurate reflection of how the patient responded to the last treatment session
D. The P portion of the note because the number of toe raises performed may be decreased in the next session

Question 85.

A PTA is teaching a family how to care for a family member at home. The patient is totally bed-bound. To prevent pressure ulcers most effectively, what should be the maximum amount of time between position changes?

A. 1 hour
B. 2 hours
C. 6 hours
D. 8 hours

Question 86.

A tennis player receives a surgical repair of the annular ligament. Where should the PTA expect to note the most edema?

A. Radial ulnar joint
B. Olecranon bursa
C. Ulnohumeral joint
D. Lateral triangle

Question 87.

A patient is referred to a therapist with a diagnosis of arthritis. What type of arthritis would the therapist expect if the patient presented with the following signs and symptoms: (1) bilateral wrists and knees are involved, (2) pain at rest and with motion, (3) prolonged morning stiffness, and (4) crepitus.

A. Osteoarthritis
B. Rheumatoid arthritis
C. Degenerative joint disease
D. It is not possible to determine with the given information.

Question 88.

A football player presents to an outpatient clinic with complaints of pain in the right knee after an injury suffered the night before. The physician determines that the anterior cruciate ligament (ACL) is torn. Which of the following is most commonly associated with an injury causing damage to the ACL only?

A. Varus blow to the knee with the foot planted and an audible pop
B.. Foot planted, medial tibial rotation, and an audible pop
C. Valgus blow to the knee with the foot planted and no audible pop
D. Foot planted, lateral tibial rotation, and no audible pop

Question 89.

A 13-year-old girl has fractured her left patella during a volleyball game. The physician determines that the superior pole is the location of the fracture. Which of the following should be avoided in early rehabilitation?

A. Full knee extension
B. 45° of knee flexion
C. 90° of knee flexion
D. 15° of knee flexion

Question 90.

A 67-year-old woman with a diagnosis of right shoulder adhesive capsulitis is evaluated by a physical therapist. The physical therapist plans to focus mostly on gaining abduction ROM. In which direction should the therapist assistant mobilize the shoulder to gain abduction ROM?

A. Posteriorly
B. Anteriorly
C. Inferiorly
D. Superiorly

Question 91.

In the geriatric population, _____ *usually* occurs after _____ is present.

A. Spondylolisthesis, spondylolysis
B. Spondylolysis, spondylolisthesis
C. Spondyloschisis, spondylolysis
D. Spondylolisthesis, spondyloschisis

Question 92.

Which of the following is not an example of a synarthrodial joint in the body?

A. Coronal suture
B. The fibrous joint between the shaft of the tibia and fibula
C. Symphysis pubis
D. Metacarpophalangeal

Question 93.

After performing an evaluation, a physical therapist notes the following information: severe spasticity of plantar flexors in the involved lower extremity; complete loss of active dorsiflexion in the involved lower extremity; and minimal spasticity between 0° and 5° of dorsiflexion, with increased spasticity when the ankle is taken into more than 5° of dorsiflexion. A PTA is consulted for application of the proper ankle-foot orthosis (AFO). Which AFO is most likely contraindicated for this patient, an 87-year-old man who had a stroke 4 weeks ago?

A. Dorsiflexion spring assist AFO
B. Posterior leaf spring AFO
C. Hinged AFO
D. Spiral AFO

Question 94.

Which of the following theories supports the use of TENS unit for sensory level pain control?

A. Gate control theory
B. Sensory interaction theory
C. Central summation theory
D. None of the above

Question 95.

A 35-year-old woman is being treated in the subacute unit of a hospital by physical, occupational, and speech therapy services for rehabilitation because of injuries suffered in a motor vehicle accident. The physical therapist and the assistant have focused on increasing the level of function of the right upper extremity. The patient's left upper extremity has full ROM and strength. The right upper extremity shoulder ROM was assessed and is recorded as follows: active flexion = 65°; passive flexion = 107°; active abduction = 55°; passive abduction = 90°; active internal rotation = 70°; passive internal rotation = 77°; active external rotation = 22°; passive external rotation = 35°; active extension = 55°; passive extension = 65°; and adduction is full actively and passively. End-feels in the involved shoulder are capsular in all planes. Which of the following would be the most important portion of the patient's exercise program?

A. Active rotator cuff exercises using a light theraband as resistance
B. Stretching exercises performed by the patient into extension
C. Passive stretching provided by the therapist assistant in all planes
D. ROM pulley exercises

Question 96.

A therapist assistant's nephew, who is a prospect for a local minor league baseball team, wants an opinion about a set of exercises that he was given by a friend. What is the best way for the assistant to approach this situation?

A. The PTA should tell the nephew to make an appointment at the outpatient clinic.
B. The PTA should have the nephew fax the exercises to the clinic; then the therapist should mark through the incorrect ones.
C. The PTA should have the nephew contact his doctor for an opinion.
D. The PTA should meet with the nephew after hours and discuss the exercises.

Question 97.

A PTA is treating an acute full-thickness burn on the entire right lower extremity of a 27-year-old man. What movements need to be stressed with splinting, positioning, and exercise to avoid contractures?

A. Hip flexion, knee extension, and ankle dorsiflexion
B. Hip extension, knee flexion, and ankle plantarflexion
C. Hip extension, knee extension, and ankle dorsiflexion
D. Hip flexion, knee extension, and ankle plantarflexion

Question 98.

A therapist is evaluating a patient in the intensive care unit. The therapist notes no eye opening, no verbal response, and no motor response. On the Glasgow coma scale, what is the patient's score?

A. 0
B. 3
C. 5
D. 9

Question 99.

To decrease the risk of hypoglycemia in a patient with type I insulin-dependent diabetes, which of the following is inappropriate?

A. Eat or drink a snack high in carbohydrates 30 minutes before exercise
B. Exercise muscles that have not had an insulin injection recently
C. Eat a carbohydrate snack for each 30–45 minutes of exercise
D. Exercise at the peak time of insulin effect

Question 100.

Which of the following is the best and first treatment for a wound with black eschar over 90% of the wound bed?

A. Lidocaine
B. Dexamethasone
C. Silvadene
D. Elase

Question 101.

The use of compression stockings on the feet and ankles is contraindicated in patients with which condition?

A. Chronic venous disease
B. Recent total knee replacement
C. Burns
D. Chronic arterial disease

Question 102.

A posterior lateral herniation of the lumbar disc between vertebrae L4 and L5 most likely results in damage to which nerve root?

A. L4
B. L5
C. L4 and L5
D. L5 and S1

Question 103.

What ligament is most involved in sustaining the longitudinal arch of the foot?

A. Plantar calcaneonavicular ligament
B. Long plantar ligament
C. Plantar calcaneocuboid ligament
D. Anterior talofibular ligament

Question 104.

A PTA is treating a 15-year-old girl with exercises to strengthen the vastus medialis obliques of bilateral knees. This patient suffers from frequent patella subluxation. The PTA explains to the patient that the most frequent position causing patella subluxation or dislocation is:

A. Foot planted with the femur going into external rotation as the knee is extending
B. Foot planted with the femur going into internal rotation as the knee is extending
C. Foot planted with the femur going into internal rotation as the knee is flexing
D. Foot planted with the femur going into external rotation as the knee is flexing

Question 105.

The PTA also informs the patient in the previous question that a _____ Q angle will predispose a person to subluxation of the patella _____.

A. Large, laterally
B. Small, laterally
C. Large, medially
D. Small, medially

Question 106.

In what position should the PTA place the upper extremity to palpate the supraspinatus tendon?

A. Full abduction, full flexion, and full external rotation
B. Full abduction, full flexion, and full internal rotation
C. Full adduction, full external rotation, and full extension
D. Full adduction, full internal rotation, and full extension

Question 107.

During the opening of a patient's mouth, a palpable and audible click is discovered in the left temporomandibular joint. The physician informs the therapist assistant that the patient has an anteriorly dislocated disk. This click most likely signifies:

A. The condyle is sliding anterior to obtain normal relationship with the disk
B. The condyle is sliding posterior to obtain normal relationship with the disk
C. The condyle is sliding anterior and losing normal relationship with the disk
D. The condyle is sliding posterior and losing normal relationship with the disk

Question 108.

At what age does a human have the greatest amount of fluid in the intervertebral disc?

A. 1 year
B. 4 years
C. 7 years
D. 10 years

Question 109.

A patient presents to an outpatient clinic with weakness of the left upper extremity. The PTA notices that during exercise, the patient is weakest with the motion of external rotation. The assistant knows that several muscles are responsible for this motion. Which of the following does not contribute or contributes the least in active external rotation of the shoulder?

A. Teres minor
B. Posterior deltoid
C. Infraspinatus
D. Latissimus dorsi

Question 110.

A PTA is reviewing the chart of a patient who is in the intensive care unit of the hospital because of a recent fall. The chart indicates that the patient has seriously compromised the eighth spinal nerve as it exits the vertebral column. Where is the likely source of this injury?

A. Above C6 vertebra
B. Above C7 vertebra
C. Above T1 vertebra
D. Above T2 vertebra

Question 111.

A PTA is treating a patient with a diagnosis of lateral epicondylitis. The physical therapist includes iontophoresis, driving dexamethasone, in the treatment plan. Dexamethasone is an _____ and is administered with the _____.

A. Analgesic, anode
B. Analgesic, cathode
C. Antiinflammatory, anode
D. Antiinflammatory, cathode

Question 112.

A patient is having pain, edema, and increased warmth at the area of the lateral epicondyle of the left upper extremity. Which of the following choices would be most beneficial for treatment of this patient's condition if no other medical condition is present that would be considered a contraindication of use of ultrasound or phonophoresis?

A. Underwater ultrasound with a 1 Mhz wand head with the intensity at 1.5 watts per square centimeter
B. Phonophoresis driving hydrocortisone with a 3 Mhz wand head with the intensity at 1.5 watts per square centimeter
C. Ultrasound with the setting in the pulsed mode, with a 20% duty cycle, using a 3 Mhz wand head
D. None of the above, because ultrasound is a direct contraindication over an area of the degree of inflammation described

Question 113.

A PTA is treating a patient who has suffered a recent stroke. There is a significant lack of dorsiflexion in the involved lower extremity and a significant amount of medial/lateral ankle instability. The assistant believes that an ankle foot orthosis (AFO) would be beneficial. Which of the following is an appropriate AFO?

A. Solid AFO
B. Posterior leaf spring AFO
C. Hinged solid AFO
D. A or C

Question 114.

A PTA is dressing the wound of a diabetic patient. The patient has a decubitus ulcer on the left foot that suddenly starts bleeding profusely. The patient is alarmed but is speaking coherently. Which of the following should be the first course of action by the therapist assistant?

A. Apply direct pressure to the wound
B. Apply a tourniquet just proximal to the malleoli
C. Active EMS
D. Apply ice and elevate the left foot above the heart

Question 115.

In order to determine if an exercise session should be terminated, the patient is asked to assess level of exertion using the Borg Rating of Perceived Exertion Scale (RPE). The patient rates the level of exertion as 9 on the 6–19 scale. A rating of 9 corresponds to which of the following?

A. Very, very light
B. Very light
C. Somewhat hard
D. Hard

Question 116.

The movement of hip external rotation occurs about a _____ axis in a _____ plane.

A. Horizontal, sagittal
B. Coronal, frontal
C. Vertical, transverse
D. Sagittal, cardinal

Question 117.

A patient is sent to outpatient rehabilitation for joint mobilization. The patient has suffered injury to the left hand and now needs mobilization of the third metacarpophalangeal joint. The therapist assistant must understand that this joint is a _____ joint in order to provide appropriate mobilization.

A. Nonaxial
B. Uniaxial
C. Biaxial
D. Triaxial

Question 118.

A patient presents to a clinic with decreased tidal volume (TV). What is the most likely cause of this change in normal pulmonary function?

A. Chronic obstructive pulmonary disease
B. Restrictive lung dysfunction
C. Bronchiectasis
D. None of the above

Question 119.

A PTA is asked by a physical therapist to treat a baseball pitcher's rotator cuff isokinetically. Which isokinetic treatment is most appropriate?

A. 190°/second, 180°/second, and 240°/second
B. 30°/second, 60°/second, and 90°/second
C. 60°/second, 120°/second, and 180°/second
D. 180°/second, 240°/second, and 360°/second

Question 120.

Which of the following tests peripheral arterial involvement in a patient with complaints of calf musculature pain?

A. Claudication time
B. Homan's sign
C. Percussion test
D. None of the above

Question 121.

To effectively treat most patients with Parkinson's disease, the PTA should emphasize which proprioceptive neuromuscular facilitation (PNF) pattern for the upper extremities?

A. D2 extension
B. D2 flexion
C. D1 extension
D. D1 flexion

Question 122.

What is the most likely cause of anterior pelvic tilt during initial contact (heel strike)?

A. Weak abdominals
B. Tight hamstrings
C. Weak abductors
D. Back pain

Question 123.

A 14-year-old girl with right thoracic scoliosis is referred to physical therapy. The PTA should expect which of the following findings?

A. Left shoulder high, left scapula prominent, and right hip high
B. Left shoulder low, right scapula prominent, and left hip high
C. Right shoulder high, right scapula prominent, and right hip high
D. Right shoulder low, right scapula prominent, and left hip high

Question 124.

A PTA is instructing a patient in performing endurance activities in the acute care department of a hospital. The patient is having difficulty breathing but is alert and oriented. The PTA discovers sounds that resemble snoring during auscultation of the patient's chest. Which of the terms below best describes these sounds?

A. Rales
B. Rhonchi
C. Wheezes
D. Crackles

Question 125.

What portion of the adult knee meniscus is vascularized?

A. Outer edge
B. Inner edge
C. The entire meniscus is vascular
D. The entire meniscus is avascular

Question 126.

Which of the following is an example of a policy in a physical therapy clinic?

A. No shorts worn in the clinic
B. The correct way to accept a telephone referral
C. The clinic will open at 8:00 am
D. A and C

Question 127.

A 14-year-old boy has suffered a traumatic brain injury resulting from a motor vehicle accident. The boy now has right lower extremity weakness, especially in the right hip abductor muscle group. The boy is anxious to recover and asks the PTA to place a 2-pound ankle weight on the involved lower extremity during sidelying right hip abduction exercise instead of using no weight. The assistant hesitates because the hip abduction strength is 3-/5 with manual muscle testing. Which of the following is a true statement?

A. A 2-pound ankle weight would assist in returning full right hip abduction active ROM more quickly than exercising without a weight.
B. A 2-pound ankle weight would cause a slower return in full right hip abduction active ROM than exercising without a weight.
C. A 1-pound weight would assist in returning full right hip abduction active ROM more quickly than exercising with a 2-pound weight or exercising without a weight.
D. B and C

Question 128.

A PTA is fitting a patient with axillary crutches. The patient has a pair of crutches that are equipped with axillary pads. The therapist assistant is fitting the patient in a standing position with the tips approximately 6 inches anteriorly and laterally to the feet. The elbows are in 20° of flexion, and the top of the axillary pads are touching the axilla. Which of the above is incorrect when fitting a person with crutches?

A. Elbows flexed at 20°
B. Crutch tips 6 inches anteriorly and laterally to the feet
C. Axilla touching the axillary pads
D. None are incorrect

Question 129.

A patient with a diagnosis of a rotator cuff tear has just begun active ROM. The therapist assistant is strengthening the rotator cuff muscles to increase joint stability and oppose the superior shear of the deltoid. Which of the rotator cuff muscles participate least in opposing the superior shear force of the deltoid?

A. Infraspinatus
B. Subscapularis
C. Teres minor
D. Supraspinatus

Question 130.

Which of the following neural fibers are the largest and fastest?

A. C fibers
B. A fibers
C. A and C are equal
D. None of the above

Question 131.

A PTA is treating a 16-year-old boy who has a diagnosis of cystic fibrosis. The therapist assistant has given the patient the following instructions: (1) take three deep breaths, (2) after you take the third breath, attempt to cough with your mouth open. Which of the following techniques is being taught by the therapist assistant?

A. Huffing
B. Controlled coughing
C. Splinted coughing
D. Pacing

Question 132.

When ordering a customized wheelchair for a patient, the physical therapist determines that the pelvic belt needs to be positioned so that it allows active anterior pelvic tilt. The PTA is asked to order the wheelchair. What is the best position for the pelvic belt in relation to the sitting surface?

A. 30°
B. 45°
C. 60°
D. 90°

Question 133.

A PTA is working in a cardiac rehabilitation setting. Which of the following types of exercises are most likely to be harmful to a 64-year-old man with a history of myocardial infarction?

A. Concentric
B. Eccentric
C. Aerobic
D. Isometric

Question 134.

A 42-year-old receptionist presents to an outpatient physical therapy clinic complaining of low back pain. The physical therapist decides that postural modification needs to be part of the treatment plan. What is the best position for the lower extremities while the patient is sitting?

A. 90° of hip flexion, 90° of knee flexion, and 10° of dorsiflexion
B. 60° of hip flexion, 90° of knee flexion, and 0° of dorsiflexion
C. 110° of hip flexion, 80° of knee flexion, and 10° of dorsiflexion
D. 90° of hip flexion, 90° of knee flexion, and 0° of dorsiflexion

Question 135.

What is the closed-packed position of the shoulder?

A. Internal rotation and abduction
B. External rotation and abduction
C. Internal rotation and adduction
D. External rotation and adduction

Question 136.

In an attempt to establish a home exercise program, the PTA gives a patient written exercises. After 1 week, the patient returns and has not performed any of the exercises. After further questioning, the assistant determines that the patient is illiterate. What is the best course of action?

A. Go over the exercises in a one-on-one review session
B. Give the patient a picture of the exercises
C. Give a copy of the exercises to a literate family member
D. All of the above

Question 137.

A PTA is working in a nursing home. The company for which the assistant works requires that employees be at least 75% efficient. The assistant realizes that he or she cannot effectively treat the patients in the given time frame. What is the best course of action?

A. Work until the 75% limit is up and cease treatment.
B. Work with the patients until the 75% limit is up and complete paperwork for the rest of the 8-hour working day.
C. Quit the job and find a company that does not require the 75% limit.
D. Go to the immediate supervisor in an attempt to alleviate the problem.

Question 138.

A home health physical therapist assistant arrives late at the home of a patient for a treatment session just as the occupational therapist has finished. The patient is angry because the sessions are so close together. The patient becomes verbally abusive toward the assistant. The most appropriate response to the patient is:

A. "I'm sorry I'm late, but you must try to understand that I am extremely busy."
B. "I know you are aggravated. It is inconvenient when someone does not show up when expected. Let's just do our best this session, and I will make an effort to see that we do not have PT and OT scheduled so close together from now on."
C. "You have to expect visits at any time of the day with home health."
D. "The occupational therapist and I did not purposefully come so close together. I apologize. Please, let's begin therapy now."

Question 139.

An <u>87</u>-year-old woman presents to an outpatient physical therapy clinic complaining of pain in the left sacroiliac (SI) joint. The physical therapist has suggested SI mobilization techniques. The examination reveals higher left anterior superior iliac spine (ASIS) than right anterior superior iliac spine (ASIS), shorter leg length on the left side (measured in supine position), and the left side posterior superior iliac spine (PSIS) lower than the right posterior superior iliac spine (PSIS). In what position should you place the patient to perform the correct sacroiliac mobilization of the left innominate?

A. Right sidelying
B. Supine
C. Prone
D. None of the above

Question 140.

At what point in the gait cycle is the center of gravity the lowest?

A. Double support
B. Terminal swing
C. Deceleration
D. Mid-stance

Question 141.

A therapist assistant is treating a 24-year-old woman who was involved in a motor vehicle accident 2 weeks ago. During the accident, the patient suffered a pneumothorax, fractured left femur, and numerous other injuries. The patient is being treated on a tilt table in an effort to increase upright tolerance. The physician has also ordered that the patient be non–weight bearing on the left lower extremity. The therapist is attempting to assist the patient in bearing weight in an upright position on the right lower extremity as soon as the table is close to a vertical position. Which of the following statements is correct?

A. It is not possible to accomplish this goal with the use of a tilt table.
B. Weight bearing is possible using a tilt table, but a minimum of 50% body weight will be placed on each lower extremity.
C. A block should be placed under the left foot.
D. None of the above

Question 142.

A physical therapist receives an order to evaluate and treat a 76-year-old woman who was involved in a motor vehicle accident 2 days ago. The patient's vehicle was struck in the rear by another vehicle. The patient has normal sensation and strength in bilateral lower extremities but paralysis and loss of sensation in bilateral upper extremities. Bowel and bladder function are normal. The patient most likely has what type of spinal cord injury?

A. Anterior cord syndrome
B. Brown-Sequard syndrome
C. Central cord syndrome
D. There is no evidence of an incomplete spinal cord lesion

Question 143.

A PTA is ambulating a 42-year-old man who has just received an above-knee prosthesis for the left leg. The assistant notices pistoning of the prosthesis as the patient ambulates. Which of the following is the most probable cause of this deviation?

A. The socket is too small.
B. The socket is too large.
C. The foot bumper is too soft.
D. The foot bumper is too hard.

Question 144.

A PTA begins treatment on a patient with a boutonnière deformity. With this injury, the involved finger usually presents in the position of:

A. Flexion of the proximal interphalangeal (PIP) joint and flexion of the distal interphalangeal (DIP) joint
B. Extension of the PIP joint and flexion of the DIP joint
C. Flexion of the PIP joint and extension of the DIP joint
D. Extension of the PIP joint and extension of the DIP joint

Question 145.

A physical therapist and a PTA are working together with a patient who has received a total knee replacement 2 days earlier. The physician has ordered application of a continuous passive machine (CPM) to the involved lower extremity. The order states that the patient should have the CPM in place throughout the entire night but has ordered no specific settings. The therapist is able to assist the patient in achieving 65° of knee flexion passively with maximum effort after approximately 30 minutes of passive ROM provided by the therapist. The therapist then places the involved lower extremity in the CPM and sets the machine to full knee extension and _____ knee flexion. Fill in the blank with the most appropriate knee flexion setting, assuming the machine is actually achieving the setting applied.

A. 90°
B. 55°
C. 65°
D. 75°

Question 146.

If the line of gravity is posterior to the hip joint in standing, on what does the body first rely to keep the trunk from moving into excessive lumbar extension?

A. Iliopsoas muscle activity
B. Abdominal muscle activity
C. Anterior pelvic ligaments and the hip joint capsule
D. Posterior pelvic ligaments and the hip joint capsule

Question 147.

Which of the following is observed by the PTA if a patient is correctly performing an anterior pelvic tilt in standing position?

A. Hip extension and lumbar flexion
B. Hip flexion and lumbar extension
C. Hip flexion and lumbar flexion
D. Hip extension and lumbar extension

Question 148.

A patient presents to physical therapy with complaints of pain in the right hip caused by osteoarthritis (OA). Which of the following is not true about this type of arthritis?

A. It causes pain usually symmetrically because it is a systemic condition.
B. It is not usually more painful in the morning.
C. This type of arthritis commonly involves the distal interphalangeal joint.
D. It mainly involves weight-bearing joints.

Question 149.

What is the best way to first exercise the postural (or extensor) musculature when it is extremely weak to facilitate muscle control?

A. Isometrically
B. Concentrically
C. Eccentrically
D. Isokinetically

Question 150.

A physical therapist is examining a 3-year-old child who is positioned as follows: supine, hips flexed to 90°, hips fully adducted, and knees flexed. The therapist passively abducts and raises the thigh, applying an anterior shear force to the hip joints. A click at 30° of abduction is noted by the therapist. What orthopedic test is the therapist performing, and what is its significance?

A. Ortolani's test—hip dislocation
B. Appley's compression/distraction test—cartilage damage
C. McMurray test—cartilage damage
D. Piston test—hip dislocation

Question 151.

A PTA is crutch training a 26-year-old man who underwent right knee arthroscopy 10 hours ago. The patient's weight-bearing status is toe-touch weight bearing on the right lower extremity. If the patient is going up steps, which of the following is the correct sequence of verbal instructions?

A. "Have someone stand below you while going up, bring the left leg up first, and then bring up the crutches and the right leg."
B. "Have someone stand above you while going up, bring the left leg up first, and then bring up the crutches and the right leg."
C. "Have someone stand below you while going up, bring the right leg up first, and then bring up the crutches and the left leg."
D. "Have someone stand above you while going up, bring the right leg up first, and then bring up the crutches and the right leg."

Question 152.

A patient's lawyer calls the PTA requesting his client's clinical records. The lawyer states that he needs the records in order to pay the patient's bill. What is the best course of action by the therapist assistant?

A. Tell the lawyer either to have the patient request a copy of the records or have the patient sign a medical release.
B. Fax the needed chart to the lawyer.
C. Mail a copy of the chart to the patient.
D. Call the patient and tell him or her of the recent development.

Question 153.

While observing a patient with posttraumatic brain injury (TBI), a PTA notes an increase in left ankle plantarflexion during loading response (heel strike to foot flat) of the involved lower extremity. With this particular patient, the left side is the involved side. Which of the following is not a likely cause of this deviation?

A. Spasticity of the left gastrocnemius
B. Hypotonicity of the left tibialis anterior
C. Leg length discrepancy
D. Left quadricep hypertonicity

Question 154.

A mother comes to a PTA concerned that her 4-month-old infant cannot yet sit up alone. Which of the following responses is the most appropriate for the assistant?

A. "Your infant probably needs further evaluation by a specialist because, although it varies, infants can usually sit up unsupported at 2 months of age."
B. "Your infant probably needs further evaluation by a specialist because, although it varies, infants can usually sit up unsupported at 3 months of age."
C. "This is probably nothing to be concerned about because, although it varies, most infants can sit up unsupported at 8 months of age."
D. "This is probably nothing to be concerned about because, although it varies, most infants can sit up unsupported at 5 months at age."

Question 155.

The protocol for a cardiac patient states that the patient should not exceed 5 METs with any activity at this stage of recovery. Which of the following activities would be inappropriate for this patient?

A. Cycling 11 mph
B. Walking 4 mph
C. Driving a car
D. Weeding a garden

Question 156.

A patient is referred to a PTA after being evaluated by a physical therapist. The patient presents with complaints of pain in the groin area (along the medial left thigh). With manual muscle testing of the involved lower extremity a therapist determines the following: hip flexion = 4+/5; hip extension = 4+/5; hip abduction = 4+/5; hip adduction = 2+/5; hip internal rotation = 2+/5; and hip external rotation = 2+/5. Which nerve on the involved side is most likely injured?

A. Lateral cutaneous nerve of the upper thigh
B. Obturator nerve
C. Femoral nerve
D. Ilioinguinal nerve

Question 157.

A PTA is treating a patient with left-side visual field deficits in both eyes. A lesion at what location may cause this deficit?

A. At the optic chiasm
B. At the right side optic tract
C. At the left side optic nerve
D. At the right side optic nerve

Question 158.

A PTA routinely places ice on the ankle of a patient with an acute ankle sprain. Ice application has many therapeutic benefits. Which of the following is the body's first response to application of ice?

A. Vasoconstriction of local vessels
B. Decreased nerve condition velocity
C. Decreased local sensitivity
D. All occur simultaneously

Question 159.

A PTA is applying mechanical traction to a patient who is having pain as a result of a nerve root being compressed as it exits the intervertebral foramen. The assistant knows from this information alone that positioning the spine in which of the following positions would be most beneficial for this patient?

A. The involved spinal area positioned in flexion
B. The involved spinal area positioned in neutral
C. The involved spinal area positioned in extension
D. The spinal area should be positioned in the same manner as that of a patient who needs maximum separation of the disk space

Question 160.

A physician notes a vertebral fracture in the radiograph of a patient involved in a car accident. The fractured vertebra has a bifid spinous process. Which of the following vertebrae is the most likely to be involved?

A. Fourth lumbar vertebra
B. Fifth cervical vertebra
C. Twelfth thoracic vertebra
D. First sacral vertebra

Question 161.

A patient presents to an outpatient physical therapy clinic with a severed ulnar nerve of the right upper extremity. What muscle is still active and largely responsible for the obvious hyperextension at the metacarpophalangeal (MCP) joints of the involved hand?

A. Dorsal interossei
B. Volar interossei
C. Extensor carpi radialis brevis
D. Extensor digitorum

Question 162.

A physical therapist assistant is attempting to find the age-adjusted maximum heart rate of a 42-year-old man. Which of the following would be the correct method to use?

A. $(220–42) \times 0.60$
B. $(220–42) \times 0.80$
C. $220–42$
D. $(220 + 42) \times 0.75$

Question 163.

A PTA is ordered to treat a patient in the intensive care unit. The patient appears to be in a coma and is totally unresponsive to noxious, visual, and auditory stimuli. What rating on the Rancho Los Amigos Cognitive Functioning Scale is most appropriate?

A. I
B. III
C. IV
D. VIV

Question 164.

A 55-year-old man is receiving instruction on how to descend stairs with a standard straight cane as an assistive device. The patient has an injured left ankle that is painful and slightly unstable. The stairs have a handrail on the right side (when descending). Which of the following statements is correct?

A. The patient should initially lower the right leg after the cane.
B. The patient should initially lower the cane and then the left leg.
C. The patient should lower the cane and the right leg together.
D. The rail should not be used, and the cane should be in the right hand.

Question 165.

A patient reports to therapy stating that his "sugar is too high" for exercise. What is the minimal blood glucose level that is considered too high for a diabetic patient to begin exercise?

A. 300 mg/dL
B. 400 mg/dL
C. 300 mg/dL
D. 400 mg/dL

Question 166.

A PTA is treating a patient in an outpatient facility for strengthening of bilateral lower extremities. During the initial treatment, the patient reveals that he has a form of cancer but is reluctant to offer any other information about his medical history. After 1 week of treatment, the assistant is informed by the physician that the patient has Kaposi's sarcoma and AIDS. Which of the following is the best course of action for the therapist?

A. Cease treatment of the patient and inform him that an outpatient facility is not the appropriate environment for a person with his medical condition.
B. Continue treatment of the patient in the gym, avoiding close contact with other patients and taking appropriate universal precautions.
C. Continue treatment of the patient in the gym as before, taking appropriate universal precautions.
D. Cease treatment, but do not confront the patient with the knowledge of his AIDS status.

Question 167.

A 25-year-old woman has been evaluated by a physical therapist and referred to a PTA because of low back pain. The PTA is performing an ultrasound at the L3 paraspinal level (which is within the plan of care) when the patient suddenly informs the assistant that she is looking forward to having her third child. On further investigation, the assistant discovers that the patient is in the first trimester of pregnancy. Which of the following is the best course of action for the assistant?

A. Change the settings of the ultrasound from continuous to pulsed.
B. Continue with the continuous setting because first-trimester pregnancy is not a contraindication.
C. Cease treatment, notify the supervising therapist, and document the mistake.
D. Send the patient to the gynecologist for an immediate sonogram.

Question 168.

Which of the following assistive devices are the most stable, and which requires the most coordination: standard walker, hemiwalker, straight cane, forearm crutches, rolling walker, quad cane, and axillary crutches?

A. The rolling walker is the most stable, and the quad cane requires the most coordination.
B. Axillary crutches are the most stable and require the most coordination.
C. The standard walker is the most stable, and axillary crutches require the most coordination.
D. None of the above

Question 169.

What lobe of the lungs is the PTA attempting to drain if the patient is in the following position: resting on the left side, rolled 1/4 turn back, supported with pillows, and the foot of the bed raised 12 to 16 inches.

A. Right middle lobe, lingular segment
B. Left upper lobe, lingular segment
C. Right upper lobe, posterior segment
D. Left upper lobe, posterior segment

Question 170.

A patient is receiving instruction on how to transfer from sitting to standing using a chair with arm rests. The physical therapist assistant erroneously provides the following instructions: (1) scoot forward in the chair, (2) place your feet shoulder width apart, (3) pull your feet back so they are behind your knees (close to the front edge of the chair), (4) do not lean forward or back (with the upper trunk) when standing, and (5) use the arm rests to help you push up to a standing position. Which of the above information is incorrect?

A. Scoot forward in the chair.
B. Place your feet shoulder width apart.
C. Pull your feet back so that they are behind your knees (close to the front edge of the chair).
D. Do not lean forward or back (with the upper trunk) when standing.

Question 171.

A PTA is monitoring a patient as she exercises on an upper extremity cycle. The patient has no particular complaints or unusual signs, but the assistant decides to assess the patient's blood pressure. The diastolic pressure is found to be 132 mm Hg. Which of the following statements is correct?

A. The diastolic pressure is represented by the top number when recording a person's blood pressure. The exercise session of this patient should continue.
B. The diastolic pressure is represented by the bottom number when recording a person's blood pressure. The exercise session of this patient should be stopped.
C. The diastolic pressure is represented by the top number when recording a person's blood pressure. The exercise session of this patient should be stopped.
D. The diastolic pressure is represented by the bottom number when recording a person's blood pressure. The exercise session of this patient should continue.

Question 172.

A PTA is treating a patient with a T4 spinal cord injury when the patient suddenly complains of a severe headache. The assistant also notes that the patient's pupils are constricted and that the patient is sweating profusely. Which of the following is the best course of action for the therapist assistant?

A. Try to find a probable source of noxious stimulus and position the patient supine with the feet elevated.
B. Try to find a probable source of noxious stimulus and position the patient with upper trunk elevated and legs lowered.
C. Try to find a probable source of noxious stimulus and place the patient in a sidelying position.
D. Try to find a probable source of noxious stimulus and position the patient in a prone position.

Question 173.

A PTA should place the knee in which of the following positions to palpate the lateral collateral ligament (LCL)?

A. Knee at 60° of flexion and the hip externally rotated
B. Knee at 20° of flexion and the hip at neutral
C. Knee at 90° of flexion and the hip externally rotated
D. Knee at 0° and the hip at neutral

Question 174.

The PTA is treating a track athlete who specializes in sprinting and wants to increase his or her speed on the track. To accomplish this goal, the plan of care should include activities to develop fast-twitch muscle fibers. Characteristics of this type fiber include:

A. Fatigues slowly, fiber colors appear red, and used more in aerobic activity
B. Fatigues quickly, fiber colors appear white, and used in anaerobic activity
C. Fatigues quickly, fiber colors appear white, and used more in aerobic activity
D. Fatigues slowly, fiber colors appear white, and used more in anaerobic activity

Question 175.

A PTA is preparing to apply intermittent compression to a new patient. The assistant is reviewing the plan of care provided by the supervising physical therapist and notices that this modality is indicated for this patient who has _____.

A. Edema in bilateral lower extremities caused by obstructed lymph vessels
B. Edema in the left lower extremity caused by infected knee joint
C. Edema in bilateral lower extremities caused by venous insufficiency
D. Edema in bilateral lower extremities and kidney dysfunction

Question 176.

Which of the following duties cannot be legally performed by a PTA?

A. Confer with a doctor about a patient's status
B. Add 5 pounds to a patient's current exercise protocol
C. Allow a patient to increase in frequency from 2 times/week to 3 times/week
D. Perform joint mobilization

Question 177.

A PTA is reviewing the chart of a new outpatient. The assistant first notices information in the chart that was provided by the patient's caregiver, because the patient is unable to verbalize his condition or surroundings. The assistant notes that the patient's home is small with little room to negotiate with a standard walker. The assistant also notes that the patient has carpet throughout the house and many throw rugs. If the initial assessment is written in SOAP note form, in which of the following should the assistant have found the above information?

A. The S portion
B. The O portion
C. The A portion
D. The P portion

Question 178.

A PTA is applying ice to a patient secondary to an ankle sprain. Of the following information, which would be incorrect to convey to this patient?

A. Muscle spindle activity decreases during cryotherapy.
B. Nerve conduction velocity decreases during cryotherapy.
C. Muscle viscosity decreases during cryotherapy.
D. Local metabolism decreases during cryotherapy.

Question 179.

A PTA has given a patient an ultraviolet treatment. The patient calls the assistant the next day with complaints of peeling and itching. These signs and symptoms resolve 3 days later (a total of 4 days after the treatment). What dose did the patient receive?

A. Suberythemal dose
B. Minimal erythemal dose
C. First-degree erythemal dose
D. Third-degree erythemal dose

Question 180.

While observing the gait pattern of a 57-year-old man with an arthritic right hip, a PTA observes a right lateral trunk lean. Why does the patient present with this gait deviation?

A. To move weight toward the involved hip and increase joint compression force
B. To move weight toward the uninvolved hip and decrease joint compression force
C. To bring the line of gravity closer to the involved hip joint
D. To take the line of gravity away from the involved hip joint

Question 181.

A PTA is mobilizing a patient's right shoulder. The movement taking place at the joint capsule is not completely to end range. It is a large-amplitude movement from near the beginning of available range to near the end of available range. What grade mobilization, according to Maitland, is being performed?

A. Grade I
B. Grade II
C. Grade III
D. Grade IV

Question 182.

A patient recently diagnosed with multiple sclerosis presents to a physical therapy clinic. The patient asks the PTA what she needs to avoid with this condition. Which of the following should the patient avoid?

A. Hot tubs
B. Slightly increased intake of fluids
C. Application of ice packs
D. Strength training

Question 183.

Which of the following actions places the greatest stress on the patellofemoral joint?

A. When the foot first contacts the ground during the gait cycle
B. Exercising on a stair-stepper machine
C. Running down a smooth decline of 30°
D. Squats to 120° of knee flexion

Question 184.

A PTA in an outpatient clinic is scheduled to continue treatment on an already established patient with a diagnosis of plantar fasciitis. Upon arrival to the clinic, the patient presents a physician's order to begin treatment of an acute second-degree ankle sprain that he suffered yesterday. The patient wishes to begin immediate treatment for the ankle sprain. What is the best course of action by the PTA?

A. Begin ice and compression on the ankle.
B. Give the patient crutches and instruct him in partial weight-bearing ambulation.
C. Contact the referring physician for advice.
D. Inform the supervising therapist of the new order before beginning any treatment.

Question 185.

On examination of a cross-section of the spinal cord of a cadaver, the examiner notes plaques. This finding is most characteristic of which condition?

A. Parkinson's disease
B. Myasthenia gravis
C. Multiple sclerosis
D. Dementia

Question 186.

A supervising physical therapist instructs a PTA to begin continuous lumbar traction on a 62-year-old woman who weighs 147-pounds. This particular patient has a diagnosis of L2 disc herniation. Through conversation with the patient, the assistant learns that she has a history of rheumatoid arthritis. What is the best course of action by the assistant?

A. Follow the treatment plan set by the physical therapist.
B. Consult with the supervising therapist because rheumatoid arthritis is a contraindication.
C. Apply intermittent traction instead of continuous traction.
D. Use continuous traction with the weight setting at 110 pounds.

Question 187.

Which of the following muscles must contract to maintain erect stance if the line of gravity (as viewed laterally) falls anterior to the lateral malleolus and anterior to the knee?

A. Gastrocnemius and quadriceps
B. Gastrocnemius and hamstrings
C. Anterior tibialis and quadriceps
D. Anterior tibialis and hamstrings

Question 188.

A PTA is treating a 32-year-old woman for complaints of right hip pain. The patient has injured the strongest ligament of the hip. The assistant places the patient in the prone position on the plinth and passively extends the involved hip. The PTA notes an abnormal amount of increase in passive hip extension. Which of the following ligaments is damaged?

A. Ischiofemoral ligament
B. Iliofemoral ligament (Y ligament of Bigelow)
C. Pubofemoral ligament
D. Ligamentum teres

Question 189.

A pitcher is exercising in a clinic with a sports cord mounted behind and above his head. The pitcher simulates the pitching motion using the sports cord as resistance. Which proprioceptive neuromuscular facilitation (PNF) diagonal is the pitcher using to strengthen the muscles involved in pitching a baseball?

A. D1 extension
B. D1 flexion
C. D2 extension
D. D2 flexion

Question 190.

A PTA is beginning treatment on a patient with an acute second-degree anterior talofibular ligament ankle sprain. Which of the following motions should be avoided in early active ROM exercises?

A. Plantarflexion and inversion
B. Plantarflexion and eversion
C. Dorsiflexion and inversion
D. Dorsiflexion and eversion

Question 191.

Which of the following positions would be the most stressful to a patient who has recently suffered a posterior bulge of the fourth lumbar vertebral disc?

A. Standing upright with the feet shoulders width apart
B. Supine with the pelvis in a neutral position
C. Standing with the lumbar spine in 90° of flexion
D. Sidelying with the knees and hips flexed to 90°

Question 192.

What is the major concern of a PTA assistant treating a patient with an acute deep partial-thickness burn covering 27% of the total body? The patient was admitted to the intensive care burn unit 2 days ago.

A. ROM
B. Fluid retention
C. Helping the family cope with the injured patient
D. Home modifications on discharge

Question 193.

A PTA is treating a 52-year-old woman after right total hip replacement. The patient complains of being self-conscious about a limp. She carries a heavy briefcase to and from work every day. The PTA notes a Trendelenburg gait during ambulation on level surfaces. What advice can the assistant give the patient to minimize this gait deviation?

A. Carry the briefcase in the right hand.
B. Carry the briefcase in the left hand.
C. Do not carry a briefcase at all.
D. It does not matter in which hand the briefcase is carried.

Question 194.

A PTA is treating a baseball pitcher who will be discharged from outpatient rehabilitation within the next week. The physical therapist has begun sport specific exercises with this patient. Which of the following would be the most challenging exercise for this patient?

A. Isotonic exercise
B. Isometric exercise
C. Concentric exercise
D. Plyometric exercise

Question 195.

Which of the following is a contraindication to ultrasound at 1.5 watts/cm^2 with a 1-MHz sound head?

A. Over a recent fracture site
B. Over noncemented metal implant
C. Over a recently surgically repaired tendon
D. Over the quadriceps muscle belly

Question 196.

While ambulating a stroke patient (the right side is the involved side), a PTA notes increased circumduction of the right lower extremity. Which of the following is an unlikely cause of this deviation?

A. Increased spasticity of the right gastrocnemius
B. Increased spasticity of the right quadriceps
C. Weak hip flexors
D. Weak knee extensors

Question 197.

A PTA is treating a patient that has a Salter-Harris fracture. This patient is most likely a
_____.

A. 12-year-old boy
B. 25-year-old woman
C. 50-year-old man
D. 90-year-old woman

Question 198.

A PTA is instructed to provide electrical stimulation to a patient with a venous stasis ulcer on the right lower extremity. What is the correct type of electrical stimulation to promote wound healing?

A. Biphasic pulsed current
B. Direct current
C. Interferential current
D. Transcutaneous electrical stimulation

Question 199.

A PTA is asked by the supervising therapist to treat a 12-year-old boy with a diagnosis of patella tendonitis. The supervising therapist has suggested eccentric quadriceps strengthening, hamstring stretching, ultrasound, and ice. Which of the suggested treatments should be avoided with this patient?

A. Eccentric quadriceps strengthening
B. Hamstring stretching
C. Ultrasound
D. Ice

Question 200.

A patient consults a PTA because of a pronounced tuft of hair on the center of her spinal column in the lumbar area. The assistant notes no loss in motor or sensory function. This patient most likely has what form of spina bifida?

A. Meningocele
B. Meningomyelocele
C. Spina bifida occulta
D. None of the above

Question 201.

While observing the standing posture of a patient, a PTA notes that a spinous process in the thoracic region is shifted laterally. This assistant estimates that T2 is the involved vertebra because he notes that it is at the approximate level of the:

A. Inferior angle of the scapula
B. Superior angle of the scapula
C. Spine of the scapula
D. Xiphoid process of the sternum

Question 202.

A PTA is testing key muscles on a patient who recently suffered a spinal cord injury. The current test assesses the strength of the long toe extensors. Which nerve segment primarily innervates this key muscle group?

A. L2
B. L3
C. L4
D. L5

Question 203.

A PTA is ambulating a patient with an above-knee amputation. The new prosthesis causes the heel on the involved foot to move laterally at toe-off. Which of the following is the most likely cause of this deviation?

A. Too much internal rotation of the prosthetic knee
B. Too much external rotation of the prosthetic knee
C. Too much outset of prosthetic foot
D. None of the above would cause this deviation

Question 204.

A 31-year-old woman with a diagnosis of lateral epicondylitis is receiving ultrasound. Which of the following is true concerning the frequency of ultrasound in this application?

✓ A. 3.0 MHz should be used
B. 1.0 MHz should be used
C. 3.0 MHz and 1.0 MHz are equally as effective
D. Ultrasound is contraindicated for this diagnosis

Question 205.

A 68-year-old man is being treated by a PTA after a right below-knee amputation. The patient is beginning ambulation with a preparatory prosthesis. In the early stance phase of the involved lower extremity, the assistant notes an increase in knee flexion. Which of the following are possible causes of this gait deviation?

A. The heel is too stiff.
B. The foot is set too far anterior in relation to the knee.
C. The foot is set in too much plantarflexion.
D. All of the above

Question 206.

When comparing the gait cycle of young adults with the gait cycle of older adults, what would a therapist assistant expect to find?

A. Younger patients have a shorter step length.
B. Younger patients have a shorter stride length.
C. Younger patients have a shorter period of double support.
D. Younger patients have a decrease in speed of ambulation.

Question 207.

When the knee is at its maximal amount of flexion during the gait cycle, which of the following muscles is active concentrically?

A. Hamstrings
B. Gluteus maximus
C. Gastrocnemius
D. All of the above

Question 208.

The terms below refer to properties of water that make hydrotherapy valuable to a variety of patient populations. Match the following terms with the statement that best relates to each term.

1. Viscosity
2. Buoyancy
3. Relative density
4. Hydrostatic pressure
    a. This property can assist in prevention of blood pooling in the lower extremities of a patient in the pool above waist level.
    b. This property makes it harder to walk faster through water.
    c. A person with a higher amount of body fat can float more easily than a lean person because of this property.
    d. This property makes it easier to move a body part to the surface of the water and harder to move a part away from the surface.

A. 1-b, 2-c, 3-d, 4-a
B. 1-b, 2-d, 3-c, 4-a
C. 1-c, 2-b, 3-a, 4-d
D. 1-a, 2-c, 3-b, 4-d

Question 209.

In the terminal swing phase of gait, what muscles of the foot and ankle are active?

A. Extensor digitorum longus
B. Gastrocnemius
C. Tibialis posterior
D. B and C

Question 210.

An outpatient PTA is gait training a patient recently discharged from the hospital. The inpatient therapist's notes describe a decrease in left stride length caused by pain with weight bearing on the right lower extremity. The outpatient assistant knows that the patient's gait deviation is:

A. An abnormally short distance from the left heel strike and the successive right heel strike
B. An abnormally short amount of time between the left heel strike and the successive right heel strike
C. An abnormally short amount of time in stance phase on the left lower extremity
D. An abnormally short distance between the left heel strike and the successive left heel strike

Question 211.

What motion takes place at the lumbar spine with right lower extremity single limb support during the gait cycle?

A. Left lateral flexion
B. Right lateral flexion
C. Extension
D. Flexion

Question 212.

A PTA is scheduled to treat a patient with a chronic condition of "hammer toes." Where should the assistant expect to find callus formation?

A. The distal tips of the toes
B. The superior surface of the interphalangeal joints
C. The metatarsal heads
D. All of the above

Question 213.

A PTA begins gait training for a patient with bilateral knee flexion contractures at 30° at a long-term care facility. The therapist knows that the patient will have a forward trunk lean during gait because:

A. The patient's line of gravity is anterior to the hip.
B. The patient's line of gravity is anterior to the knee.
C. The patient's line of gravity is anterior to the ankle.
D. A and C

Question 214.

A PTA is treating a patient with diffuse ankle pain. This patient also has advanced peripheral arterial disease. Which of the following modalities should be used?

A. Ice packs
B. Hot packs
C. Continuous ultrasound
D. None of the above

Question 215.

A 43-year-old man with right biceps brachii rupture presents to physical therapy after a surgical repair. According to the surgeon, the rupture was at the musculotendinous junction. Which of the following has most likely been compromised?

A. Meissner's corpuscles
B. Merkel's disks
C. Ruffini endings
D. Golgi tendon organs

Question 216.

A PTA is treating an automobile mechanic. The patient asks for tips on preventing upper extremity repetitive motion injuries. Which of the following is incorrect advice?

A. Use your entire hand rather than just the fingers when holding an object.
B. Position tasks so they are performed below shoulder height.
C. Use tools with small, straight handles when possible.
D. When performing a forceful task, keep the materials slightly lower than the elbow.

Question 217.

A PTA is treating a patient who underwent a total knee replacement 4 weeks ago. The patient is ambulating with a rolling walker independently for functional distances and is performing all transfers independently. The current plan of care calls for quadriceps and hamstring strengthening, stretching, gait training, and ice application. Knee extension lacks 2° actively, and flexion is 110° actively. Passive ROM measures 0° to 125° in the involved knee. During straight leg raises with a 5-pound weight on the patient's ankle, a 10° quadriceps lag from neutral is noted. What is the best course of action by the PTA?

A. Contact the supervising therapist
B. Decrease the weight to 3 pounds
C. Continue with the current 5-pound weight
D. Increase the weight to at least 6 pounds

Question 218.

A PTA is speaking to a group of receptionists about correct posture. Which of the following is incorrect information?

A. Position computer monitors at eye level.
B. Position seats so that the feet are flat on the floor while sitting.
C. Position keyboards so that the wrists are in approximately 20° of extension.
D. Take frequent stretching breaks.

Question 219.

Which of the following is an inappropriate exercise for a patient who received an anterior cruciate ligament reconstruction with a patella tendon autograft 2 weeks ago?

A. Lateral step-ups
B. Heel slides
C. Stationary bike
D. Pool walking

Question 220.

When ambulating on uneven terrain, how should the subtalar joint be positioned to allow forefoot rotational compensation?

A. Pronation
B. Supination
C. Neutral position
D. The position of the subtalar joint does not influence forefoot compensation

Question 221.

A PTA is attempting to explain the importance of slow stretching to an athlete training to compete in a marathon. The assistant explains that quick stretching often causes the muscle to _____, which is a response initiated by the _____ , which are located in the muscle fibers.

A. Relax—Golgi tendon organs
B. Contract—Golgi tendon organs
C. Relax—muscle spindles
D. Contract—muscle spindles

Question 222.

A physical therapist is performing passive ROM on the shoulder of a 43-year-old woman who received a rotator cuff repair 5 weeks ago. During passive ROM, the therapist notes a capsular end feel at 95° of shoulder flexion. What should the therapist do?

A. Continue with passive ROM
B. Begin joint mobilization
C. Immediately schedule an appointment with the physician for the patient
D. A and B

Question 223.

A patient presents to outpatient physical therapy with tarsal tunnel syndrome. What nerve is involved? Where should the PTA concentrate treatment?

A. Superficial peroneal nerve—inferior to the medial malleolus
B. Posterior tibial nerve—inferior to the medial malleolus
C. Superficial peroneal nerve—inferior to the lateral malleolus
D. Posterior tibial nerve—inferior to the lateral malleolus

Question 224.

A 30-year-old woman who had a full-term infant 4 weeks ago presents to physical therapy with diastasis recti. The separation was measured by the physician and found to be 3 cm. Which of the following exercises is most appropriate to minimize the separation?

A. Sit-ups while using the upper extremities to bring the rectus abdominis to midline
B. Bridges while using the upper extremities to bring the rectus abdominis to midline
C. Dynamic lumbar stabilization exercises in quadraped position
D. Gentle head lifts in supine position while using the upper extremities to bring the rectus abdominis to midline

Question 225.

A physical therapist is ordered to fabricate a splint for a 2-month-old infant with congenital hip dislocation. The PTA is asked to assist during this procedure. In what position should the hip be placed while the patient is in the splint?

A. Flexion and adduction
B. Extension and adduction
C. Extension and abduction
D. Flexion and abduction

Question 226.

Which of the following muscle tendons most commonly sublux in patients who suffer from rheumatoid arthritis?

A. Flexor digitorum profundus
B. Extensor carpi ulnaris
C. Extensor carpi radialis longus
D. Flexor pollicis longus

Question 227.

A PTA is writing a progress note regarding a patient that recently received a total hip arthroplasty. Part of the note will include a goniometer measurement of hip flexion active ROM. After the patient is placed in supine position, where should the fulcrum of the goniometer be placed?

A. Over the iliac crest
B. Over the greater trochanter
C. Over the adductor longus muscle belly
D. Over the anterior superior iliac spine (ASIS)

Question 228.

A patient who has suffered a zone 2 rupture of the extensor tendon of the third digit presents to physical therapy. This patient had a surgical fixation of the avulsed tendon. During the period of immobilization, which of the following deformities is most likely to develop?

A. Boutonniére deformity
B. Claw hand
C. Swan neck deformity
D. Dupuytren's contracture

Question 229.

A supervising therapist inquires about a patient's progress in treatment of de Quervain's disease. The PTA will assess passive thumb abduction as part of her report to the physical therapist. Where should the fulcrum of the goniometer be placed to measure this motion with the patient's wrist in the neutral position?

A. Over the ulnar styloid process
B. Over the web space between the thumb and second digit
C. Over the radial styloid process
D. Over the lateral portion of the interphalangeal joint

Question 230.

A PTA is beginning treatment of a 75-year-old woman with increased thoracic kyphosis and anterior pelvic tilt. Which of the following exercises should be avoided with this patient?

A. Scapular retractions
B. Hip bridges in supine
C. Toe raises
D. Hip flexion strengthening

Question 231.

A patient with complaints of low back pain has been evaluated by a physical therapist. During the evaluation, the supervising therapist finds a tight iliopsoas bilaterally. Of the choices given, what should the PTA expect to find?

A. Increased lumbar lordosis and increased thoracic kyphosis
B. Decreased lumbar lordosis and decreased thoracic kyphosis
C. Decreased lumbar lordosis and increased thoracic kyphosis
D. Increased lumbar lordosis and decreased thoracic kyphosis

Question 232.

A physical therapist is performing an evaluation on a patient. The patient is supine with the arms crossed over the chest. The therapist asks the patient to perform an abdominal curl. The patient curls the upper trunk until the inferior angles of the scapulae are off the treatment table. What manual muscle testing grade should be given to this patient's abdominal musculature?

A. 5/5
B. 4/5
C. 3+/5
D. 3/5

Question 233.

A PTA is performing a weekly assessment of a patient with a diagnosis of greater trochanteric bursitis. Part of this assessment will be a manual muscle test of the hip abduction musculature. The patient is placed in sidelying position with the involved lower extremity superior. The patient is asked to abduct the hip fully, and then the PTA gives resistance over the knee in an effort to push the patient's leg back to a neutral position. The muscle group being tested is innervated by what portion of the lumbosacral plexus?

A. L1-L4
B. L2-L5
C. L3-L5
D. L4-S1

Question 234.

A PTA is treating a 34-year-old woman with a diagnosis of carpal tunnel syndrome. Part of the treatment consists of grip strengthening exercises for the flexor digitorum profundus. To isolate the flexor digitorum profundus, where should the grip dynamometer's adjustable handle be placed?

A. 1 inch from the dynamometer's nonadjustable handle
B. 3 inches from the dynamometer's nonadjustable handle
C. 1.5 inches from the dynamometer's nonadjustable handle
D. All of the above are equally effective

Question 235.

A PTA is treating a patient with balance deficits. During treatment, the assistant notes that large-amplitude changes in center of mass cause the patient to lose balance. The patient, however, can accurately compensate for small changes nearly every time a change is introduced. What muscles most likely need to be strengthened to help alleviate this dysfunction?

A. Tibialis anterior, gastrocnemius
B. Peroneus longus/brevis, tibialis posterior
C. Rectus abdominis, erector spinea
D. Iliopsoas, gluteus maximus

Question 236.

A PTA is summoned to the waiting room in an outpatient facility. Upon arrival, the PTA notes a geriatric man lying face down on the floor. As the assistant approaches the patient, which of the below choices should the therapist assess first?

A. Level of consciousness
B. Airway
C. Breathing
D. Circulation

Question 237.

A PTA is treating a 75-year-old man in cardiac rehabilitation who suffered a myocardial infarction 4 weeks ago. The patient has progressed well and has voiced an increase in functional activities at home since beginning outpatient treatment. Today he presented with the following resting vital signs before exercise: blood pressure (BP), 135/85 mm Hg; heart rate (HR), 75 bpm; and a respiratory rate (RR), 13 breaths per minute. After performing 15 minutes of aerobic activity, his vital signs are measured by the PTA and recorded as follows: BP, 155/90 mm Hg; HR 100 bpm; and RR 17 breaths per minute. What should be the next course of action by the physical therapist assistant?

A. Alert the supervising therapist.
B. Tell the patient to sit and rest for a few minutes.
C. Terminate the exercise session and send the patient to the emergency room.
D. Allow the patient to continue to exercise.

Question 238.

Which of the following is not part of the triangular fibrocartilage complex of the wrist?

A. Dorsal radioulnar ligament
B. Ulnar collateral ligament
C. Radial collateral ligament
D. Ulnar articular cartilage

Question 239.

A PTA is speaking to a group of avid tennis players. A group member asks how to prevent tennis elbow (lateral epicondylitis). Which of the following is incorrect information?

A. Primarily use the wrist and elbow extensors during a backhand stroke.
B. Begin the backhand stroke in shoulder adduction and internal rotation.
C. Use a racket that has a large grip.
D. Use a light racquet.

Question 240.

Which tendon is most commonly involved with lateral epicondylitis?

A. Extensor carpi radialis longus
B. Extensor carpi radialis brevis
C. Brachioradialis
D. Extensor digitorum

Question 241.

The supervising therapist has just finished an evaluation of a patient with a stage 2 pressure ulcer. After the evaluation, the supervising therapist tells the PTA that the wound bed is "beefy red" in appearance. What should this mean to the PTA?

A. The wound is infected.
B. The wound is too moist.
C. The wound is too dry.
D. The wound is healing well.

Question 242.

A 14-year-old girl placed excessive valgus stress to the right elbow during a fall from a bicycle. Her forearm was in supination at the moment the valgus stress was applied. Which of the following is most likely involved in this type of injury?

A. Ulnar nerve
B. Extensor carpi radialus
C. Brachioradialis
D. Annular ligament

Question 243.

A PTA is reviewing the chart of a 16-year-old boy who has received an anterior cruciate ligament reconstruction. The chart indicates that the boy has received a/an _____, which indicates to the assistant that the ligament was taken from another human and not from the patient himself.

A. Autograft
B. Xenograft
C. Heterodermic graft
D. Allograft

Question 244.

A PTA is attempting to increase a patient's functional mobility in a seated position. To treat the patient most effectively and efficiently, the following should be performed in what order?

1. Weight shifting of the pelvis
2. Isometric contractions of the lower extremity
3. Trunk ROM exercises
4. Isotonic resistance to the quadriceps

A. 1, 2, 3, 4
B. 2, 3, 1, 4
C. 4, 3, 2, 1
D. 3, 2, 1, 4

Question 245.

A patient who has suffered a recent stroke is being treated by a PTA. The patient exhibits increased extensor tone in the supine position along with an exaggerated symmetric tonic labyrinthine reflex (STLR). What is the best position to initiate flexion movements of the lower extremity?

A. Prone position
B. Sidelying position
C. Supine position
D. A and B

Question 246.

A patient who suffered a T1 complete spinal cord injury is being discharged from a rehabilitation facility. The family is being trained in prevention of decubitus ulcers. Which of the following areas would be least likely to develop a pressure ulcer?

A. Heels
B. Sacrum
C. Greater trochanter
D. Popliteal fossa

Question 247.

If the patient in the above scenario develops a grade 1 pressure ulcer over the ischial tuberosities, which of the following would not assist in the healing of these wounds?

A. Have the patient sit on a donut pad 2 to 3 hours per day.
B. Perform pressure relief every 15 to 20 minutes.
C. Have the family obtain a specialized air mattress.
D. Make sure the patient has an appropriate wheelchair cushion.

Question 248.

A patient is being treated in an outpatient facility after receiving a meniscus repair to the right knee 1 week ago. The patient has full passive extension of the involved knee but lacks 4° of full extension when performing a straight leg raise. The patient's active flexion is 110° and passive flexion is 119°. What is a common term used to describe the patient's most significant ROM deficit? What is a possible source of this problem?

A. Flexion contracture—quadriceps atrophy
B. Extension lag—joint effusion
C. Flexion lag—weak quadriceps
D. Extension contracture—tight hamstrings

Question 249.

A patient presents to therapy with an ankle injury. The physical therapist has determined that the injury is at the junction of the distal tibia and fibula. Which of the following functions most in preventing excessive external rotation and posterior displacement of the fibula?

A. Anterior inferior tibiofibular ligament
B. Posterior inferior tibiofibular ligament
C. Interosseous membrane
D. None of the above

Question 250.

A 17-year-old athlete has just received a posterior cruciate ligament reconstruction. The PTA is attempting to explain some of the characteristics of the posterior cruciate ligament. Which of the following is incorrect information?

A. The posterior cruciate ligament prevents posterior translation of the tibia on the femur.
B. Posterior bands of the posterior cruciate ligament are their tightest in full knee extension.
C. The posterior cruciate ligament is attached to the lateral meniscus and not to the medial meniscus.
D. The posterior cruciate ligament helps with medial rotation of the tibia during full knee extension with open-chain activities.

Question 251.

Which of the following observations is not true when observing a patient without foot or ankle problems in the standing position?

A. The talus is situated somewhat medially to the midline of the foot.
B. In quiet standing, the muscles surrounding the ankle joint remain silent.
C. The first and second metatarsal heads bear more weight than the fourth and fifth metatarsal heads.
D. The talus transmits weight to the rest of the bones of the foot.

Question 252.

Of the following, which is the earliest period after surgery that an 18-year-old young man who received an uncomplicated partial meniscectomy of the right knee can perform functional testing, such as a one-leg hop test, for distance?

A. 1 week after surgery
B. 2 weeks after surgery
C. 6 weeks after surgery
D. 12 weeks after surgery

Question 253.

A PTA is teaching a patient with a T3 spinal cord injury proper level surface transfer techniques. In this case, the patient will use a sliding board and transfer to the left. Which of the following is the correct set of instructions in order to perform this transfer efficiently and safely?

A. Place the board between the wheelchair and the mat. The hands are then arranged posterior to the greater trochanters. As weight is removed from the buttocks with a triceps press, the head and upper trunk are forcefully twisted to the right.
B. Place the board between the wheelchair and the mat. The hands are then arranged anterior to the greater trochanters. As weight is removed from the buttocks with a triceps press, the head and upper trunk are forcefully twisted to the right.
C. Place the board between the wheelchair and the mat. The hands are then arranged anterior to the greater trochanters. As weight is removed from the buttocks with a triceps press, the head and upper trunk are forcefully twisted to the left.
D. Place the board between the wheelchair and the mat. The hands are then arranged posterior to the greater trochanters. As weight is removed from the buttocks with a triceps press, the head and upper trunk are forcefully twisted to the left.

Question 254.

A 65-year-old woman, who suffered a stroke 18 months ago is being treated in outpatient physical therapy. She has been treated for an extended length of time and has reached a plateau in her level of progression. The physical therapist has reminded the patient that today will be her last physical therapy session. Later, she turns to the PTA and adamantly requests continuation of her physical therapy. What is the best course of action by the PTA?

A. Refer the patient to social services.
B. Alert the referring physician.
C. Inform the patient that she will no longer progress because she is too weak.
D. Inform the physical therapist of the patient's request.

Question 255.

A supervising therapist has evaluated a patient with a diagnosis of Alzheimer's disease that is now being treated by a PTA. The patient is a resident of a long-term care facility. Which of the following is the most appropriate treatment regimen for this patient?

A. Give one to two step commands, treat the patient in a crowded room to challenge attention span, and schedule appointments at the same time each day.
B. Give three to four step commands, treat the patient in a crowded room to challenge attention span, and schedule appointments at different times each day.
C. Give one to two step commands, treat the patient in a quiet room, and schedule appointments at the same time each day.
D. Give one to two step commands, treat the patient in a quiet room, and schedule appointments at different times each day.

Question 256.

A supervising therapist has treated a 21-year-old man with a partial-thickness burn over the dorsum of his hand and the fingers, using whirlpool and debridement. The supervising therapist then instructs the PTA to cover the wound with an antibiotic cream and sterile bandages. Which of the following is the correct procedure to apply a moistened sterile gauze to this wound?

A. Wrap the fingers together, as in a mitt, to maintain a sterile application.
B. Wrap each finger together, as in a mitt, then anchor the dressing with a "figure 8" over the dorsum of the hand.
C. . Wrap each finger separately then anchor the dressing with a "figure 8" over the dorsum of the hand.
D. Inform the physical therapist that this is beyond the scope of training of a PTA.

Question 257.

When using universal precautions, which of the following should be the last article of protection to be donned by the PTA?

A. Mask
B. Gown
C. Eye protection
D. Gloves

Question 258.

A patient with decreased function of the gluteus minimus is referred to physical therapy for gait training. During the exercise session, the PTA places the patient in prone position and instructs the patient to extend the hip. Knowing that the gluteus minimus is extremely weak, which of the following is most likely to happen?

A. The patient will abduct the hip more than usual when attempting to perform hip extension.
B. The patient will externally rotate the hip excessively when attempting to perform hip extension.
C. The patient will excessively flex the knee when attempting to perform hip extension.
D. The patient will not have difficulty performing straight hip extension.

Question 259.

A PTA is helping the supervising therapist who is performing an evaluation on an 86-year-old woman who recently suffered a stroke. The patient has just been transferred to the hospital from a long-term care facility. The nurse informs the therapists that the patient has a stage 2 decubitis ulcer on the sacrum. The therapists must roll the patient from supine to prone to evaluate the wound. The patient is very weak and will require maximum assistance to roll. Which of the following is the correct technique to roll this patient from supine to prone, assuming patient is being rolled to the right?

A. The patient is moved to the left edge of the bed. The left leg is then crossed over the right leg. The arms are fully adducted to the patient's side. The PTA places his hands on the patient's upper trunk and pulls the patient toward him. The head is the placed in a comfortable position at the end of the transfer.
B. The patient is moved to the right edge of the bed. The right leg is then crossed over the left leg. The arms are fully adducted to the patient's side. The PTA places his hands on the patient's upper trunk and pulls the patient toward him. The head is the placed in a comfortable position at the end of the transfer.
C. The patient is moved to the left edge of the bed. The left leg is then crossed over the right leg. The arms are fully adducted to the patient's side. The PTA places his hands on the patient's upper trunk and pushes the patient away from him. The head is the placed in a comfortable position at the end of the transfer.
D. The patient is moved to the right edge of the bed. The right leg is then crossed over the left leg. The arms are fully adducted to the patient's side. The PTA places his hands on the patient's upper trunk and pushes the patient away from him. The head is placed in a comfortable position at the end of the transfer.

Question 260.

A patient is in an outpatient facility because of an injury sustained to the right knee joint. Only the structures within the synovial cavity were compromised during the injury. Knowing this information only, the PTA is not concerned with injury to which of the following structures?

A. Patellofemoral joint
B. Anterior cruciate ligament
C. Medial meniscus
D. Femoral condyles

Question 261.

A supervising therapist has just finished an evaluation of a 23-year-old man with a diagnosis of L1 complete paraplegia. The patient has been in a rehabilitation unit for several weeks and is now ready to begin outpatient physical therapy. Part of his initial treatment will be gait training with Lofstrand (forearm) crutches. Which of the following is the correct method to fit this patient with Lofstrand crutches?

A. Have the patient stand in normal erect stance (with assistance if necessary). The hand-grips should come to the ulnar styloid process, and the cuffs should be positioned superior to the elbow.
B. Have the patient stand in normal erect stance (with assistance if necessary). The hand-grips should come to the metacarpophalangeal joints, and the cuffs should be positioned superior to the elbow.
C. Have the patient stand in normal erect stance (with assistance if necessary). The hand-grips should come to the ulnar styloid process, and the cuffs should be positioned inferior to the elbow.
D. Have the patient stand in normal erect stance (with assistance if necessary). The hand-grips should come to the metacarpophalangeal joints, and the cuffs should be positioned inferior to the elbow.

Question 262.

A PTA is instructing a patient on correct sleeping positions. This patient has no abnormalities in the spine but suffers from chronic lumbar muscle spasms. Which of the following positions of sleep for this patient would most likely place the least amount of stress on the lumbar spine?

A. Prone position with a pillow under the head
B. Supine position with a pillow under the head
C. Sidelying position with a pillow under the head and between the knees
D. A and B are equally correct

Question 263.

A 47-year-old woman is referred to physical therapy because of significant balance deficits. During the initial evaluation, the patient fails a Romberg test. What does this mean to the PTA?

A. The patient relies on ankle proprioception to maintain balance.
B. The patient relies on vestibular input to maintain balance.
C. The patient relies on muscle power to maintain balance.
D. The patient relies on visual input to maintain balance.

Question 264.

A PTA is treating an 81-year-old man with Parkinson's disease. The patient has been ambulating with a cane. He was referred to physical therapy because of a fall at home. The family reports a decrease in gait ability during the past several months. The assistant is instructed to begin gait training with a rolling walker. Which of the following is incorrect for the treatment of this patient?

A. Strengthening of the hip flexors and stretching of the gluteals
B. Slow, rhythmic rocking techniques
C. Biofeedback during ambulation
D. Prolonged passive stretching of the gastrocnemius muscle group bilaterally

Question 265.

A high-school athlete is considering whether to have an anterior cruciate ligament reconstruction. The PTA explains the importance of this ligament, especially in a person who is young and athletic. Which of the statements below is correct in describing part of the function of the anterior cruciate ligament?

A. The anterior cruciate ligament prevents excessive posterior roll of the femoral condyles during flexion of the femur at the knee joint.
B. The anterior cruciate ligament prevents excessive anterior roll of the femoral condyles during flexion of the femur at the knee joint.
C. The anterior cruciate ligament prevents excessive posterior roll of the femoral condyles during extension of the femur at the knee joint.
D. The anterior cruciate ligament prevents excessive anterior roll of the femoral condyles during extension of the femur at the knee joint.

Question 266.

Which of the following statements is true in comparing infants with Down's syndrome to infants with no known abnormalities?

A. Motor milestones are reached at the same time with both groups.
B. Postural reactions are developed in the same time frame with both groups.
C. Postural reactions and motor milestones develop slower in patients who have Down's syndrome but with the same association as with normal infants.
D. Postural reactions and motor milestones do not develop with the same association with patients who have Down's syndrome as with normal infants.

Question 267.

A PTA is treating a 67-year-old man who recently suffered a stroke. The patient's main complaint is a loss of balance. Which of the following positions would challenge his balance the most?

A. Sitting in a chair with his eyes closed
B. Sitting with the upper extremities in full shoulder flexion
C. Standing on a foam block with his eyes closed
D. Standing on a flat surface with his eyes closed

Question 268.

An athlete with chronic Achilles tendonitis has just finished an intense workout. There is no edema or warmth at the Achilles tendon. He has used heat modalities in the past to control his pain after workouts. Which of the following would be an incorrect method of heat application for this athlete immediately after his workout?

A. Hot pack
B. Full-body immersion in a hot whirlpool
C. Ultrasound
D. Warm whirlpool to the ankle only

Question 269.

A PTA has been treating a 28-year-old man, with a diagnosis of tennis elbow, 3 times a week for 3 weeks in an outpatient facility. Treatments have consisted of ultrasound (with a 3-MHz sound head at 1.5 watts per square centimeter to the lateral epicondyle of the humerus), extensor musculature stretching, job modification, and ice. The patient reports no change in pain level over the past several weeks. His strength and ROM remain the same as assessed at the initial evaluation. The supervising therapist suggests the substitution of phonophoresis (instead of ultrasound), with hydrocortisone, to the treatment plan. What changes should the PTA make to the ultrasound dosage in order to effectively administer phonophoresis?

A. Change to a 1-Mhz sound head.
B. Decrease to 1.0 watts per square centimeter.
C. Phonophoresis is contraindicated in the situation.
D. There is no need to change ultrasound dosage.

Question 270.

A PTA is treating a 35-year-old man with traumatic injury to the right hand. The patient has several surgical scars from a tendon repair performed 6 weeks ago. What is the appropriate type of masssage for the patient's scars?

A. Transverse and longitudinal
B. Circular and longitudinal
C. Transverse and circular
D. Massage is contraindicated after a tendon repair

Question 271.

Which of the following statements best describes lower extremity positioning in standing during the first 2 years of life of a child with no dysfunction?

A. Femoral anteversion, femoral external rotation, foot pronation
B. Femoral anteversion, femoral internal rotation, foot supination
C. Femoral retroversion, femoral external rotation, foot pronation
D. Femoral retroversion, femoral internal rotation, foot supination

Question 272.

Which of the following sources of stimulation is least effective in obtaining functional goals when treating an infant with decreased muscular tone?

A. Vestibular
B. Weight bearing
C. Cutaneous
D. Vibratory

Question 273.

Which of the following is inappropriate for a PTA to include in the treatment of an infant with a gestational age of 27 weeks and Down's syndrome?

A. Bottle feeding
B. Encourage sidelying position
C. Tactile stimulation with the entire hand rather than the fingertips of the examiner
D. Prone positioning

Question 274.

A patient with spinal cord injury must learn techniques of muscle substitution in order to complete transfers and functional activities. Which of the following muscles could be used by a C6 complete quadriplegic in a sitting position on a plinth with the hand lateral and posterior to the hip to attain elbow extension if the involved hand is fixed and the elbow is in a slightly flexion position?

A. Anterior deltoid and pectoralis major
B. Extensor carpi radialis longus and brevis
C. Posterior deltoid and middle deltoid
D. Triceps brachii

Question 275.

In taping an athlete's ankle prophylactically before a football game, in what position should the ankle be slightly positioned before taping to provide the most protection against an ankle sprain?

A. Inversion, dorsiflexion, abduction
B. Eversion, plantarflexion, adduction
C. Eversion, dorsiflexion, abduction
D. Inversion, plantarflexion, adduction

Question 276.

A supervising therapist has suggested mechanical lumbar traction to treat a patient with a diagnosis of lumbar disc disease. The PTA will place the patient on traction. Which of the following is an incorrect procedure for initial setup of lumbar traction if the patient is in the supine postion?

A. The top of the pelvic belt should come to the umbilicus.
B. The thoracic pads should lie on the anterior/superior chest wall.
C. The bottom of the thoracic pads should be inferior to the umbilicus.
D. The pelvic belt and thoracic pads should slightly overlap.

Question 277.

A PTA is reviewing the chart of a 24-year-old woman with a diagnosis of L2 incomplete paraplegia. The physician noted that the left quadriceps tendon reflex is 2+. What does this information relay to the assistant?

A. No active quadriceps tendon reflex
B. Slight quadriceps contraction with reflex testing
C. Normal quadriceps tendon reflex
D. Exaggerated quadriceps tendon reflex

Question 278.

Which of the following is the normal end-feel perceived by an examiner assessing wrist flexion?

A. Bone to bone
B. Soft tissue approximation
C. Tissue stretch
D. Empty

Question 279.

A PTA is attempting to open the spastic and flexed hand of a patient who has suffered a recent stroke. Which of the following does not inhibit hand opening?

A. Avoid touching the interossei.
B. Apply direct pressure to the thenar eminence.
C. Hyperextend the metacarpophalangeal (MCP) joint.
D. A and B

Question 280.

Which of the following is the most important safety aspect of mechanical cervical traction?

A. Making sure the patient has a safety cut-off switch in his or her hand
B. Making sure the poundage of traction is set correctly
C. Making sure the angle of pull is appropriate
D. Making sure the duration of the on/off cycle is correct

Question 281.

A physician requests a progress note on a patient's progress who is attending outpatient physical therapy. The PTA notes increased edema in the involved knee after today's exercise session. Which of the following would be the best clinical method to assess edema in the knee?

A. Volumetrics
B. Girth measurement
C. Subjective observation by the supervising therapist
D. Subjective observation by the PTA

Question 282.

An insurance company requires functional testing of a patient before she returns to work. Which of the following is a functional test?

A. Isokinetic testing
B. Manual muscle testing
C. Measuring the time it takes the patient to climb a flight of stairs
D. Handgrip dynamometer testing

Question 283.

A PTA is treating a patient with the diagnosis of elbow tendonitis. The therapist instructs the patient to sit in a chair, flex the involved elbow to 90°, and pronate the forearm. The therapist then resists elbow flexion by the patient. Which of the following muscles is being tested?

A. Biceps brachii
B. Brachialis
C. Brachioradialis
D. Triceps brachii

Question 284.

A supervising therapist has included interferential current stimulation to the treatment plan of a 38-year-old man. A PTA is asked to perform this procedure. How many channels will be used?

A. 1
B. 2
C. 3
D. 4

Question 285.

Considering the above question, what is the most likely goal of treatment for this patient?

A. Decrease pain.
B. Promote wound healing.
C. Increase muscle strength.
D. Decrease edema.

Question 286.

Which of the following statements about developmental motor control is incorrect?

A. Isotonic control develops before isometric control.
B. Gross motor control develops before fine motor control.
C. Eccentric movement develops before concentric movement.
D. Trunk control develops before distal extremity control.

Question 287.

A PTA begins treatment of a 78-year-old man with a stage 2 decubitis ulcer over the right greater trochanter. The supervising physical therapist has described the wound as "macerated." Which of the following wound dressings would be most appropriate?

A. A dressing to moisten the wound
B. A dressing to penetrate the eschar over the wound
C. A dressing to pull moisture from the wound
D. An antibiotic dressing

Question 288.

A PTA is treating a 76-year-old woman with left lower extremity hypotonia secondary to a recent stroke. Which of the following is an incorrect method to normalize tone?

A. Rapid irregular movements
B. Approximation
C. Prolonged stretch
D. Tactile cues

Question 289.

A 76-year-old woman received a cemented right total hip arthroplasty (THA) 24 hours ago. The surgeon documented that he used a posterolateral incision. Which of the following suggestions is inappropriate for the next 24 hours?

A. Avoid hip flexion above 30°.
B. Avoid hip adduction past midline.
C. Avoid any internal rotation.
D. Avoid abduction past 15°.

Question 290.

A PTA is treating a 5-day-old infant with cerebral palsy. The infant has an abnormal amount of extensor tone. Which of the following is correct positioning advice for the family and nursing staff?

A. Keep the infant in the supine position.
B. Keep the infant in the prone position.
C. Keep the infant in the sidelying position.
D. B and C are correct

Question 291.

A PTA is gait training a patient who suffered a myocardial infarction 2 days ago. The patient has adequately performed a warm-up routine and begins ambulation with a standard walker. During ambulation, oxygen saturation is measured at 86%. What is the most appropriate course of action by the PTA?

A. Stop ambulation immediately and measure the patient's vital signs.
B. Continue ambulation but decrease the patient's pace.
C. Continue ambulation at the current pace.
D. Stop ambulation for a moment and then continue at the current pace.

Question 292.

Which of the following is widely considered the most accurate body composition assessment?

A. Hydrostatic weighing
B. Electrical impedance
C. Anthropometric measurement
D. None of the above

Question 293.

A PTA is treating a patient in the gym of an outpatient facility. The patient notices his cousin exercising her bilateral upper extremities in the gym. The patient asks the PTA, "What is she here for?" Which of the following would be appropriate in response to this question?

A. Tell the patient what his cousin is being treated for; this is not a breach in confidentiality because they are being treated openly in the gym.
B. Tell the patient what his cousin is being treated for because they are related.
C. Tell the patient that his cousin is performing exercises to strengthen the upper extremities, but do not reveal the diagnosis.
D. Inform this patient that revealing any information on another person's condition is a breach in patient confidentiality.

Question 294.

A PTA is teaching a class in geriatric fitness and strengthening at a local gym. Which of the following is not a general guideline for exercise prescription in this patient population?

A. To increase exercise intensity, increase treadmill speed rather than the grade.
B. Start at a low intensity (2–3 METs).
C. Use machines for strength training rather than free weights.
D. Set weight resistance so that the patient can perform more than 8 repetitions before fatigue.

Question 295.

A PTA is attempting to inform a patient on how to breathe correctly while performing abdominal crunches. Which of the following statements is correct?

A. The patient should exhale while the upper trunk is descending.
B. The patient should exhale while the upper trunk is ascending.
C. The patient should inhale while the upper trunk is ascending.
D. Breathing pattern is not a significant concern when performing crunches.

Question 296.

A PTA is treating a 3-year-old patient in a clinic when the patient suddenly collapses. The assistant assesses level of consciousness, airway, breathing, and the patient's pulse. Where should the pulse of a person of this age be assessed?

A. At the brachial artery
B. At the carotid artery
C. At the femoral artery
D. At the radial artery

Question 297.

A 63-year-old woman presents to physical therapy with a diagnosis of herpes zoster. The physical therapist informs the PTA that the L5 dorsal root is involved and that a TENS unit should be used to help control the pain. Where should the TENS unit electrodes be placed?

A. Posterior thigh
B. Lateral hip or greater trochanter area
C. Anterior thigh
D. Anterior lateral tibia

Question 298.

A PTA is reviewing the chart of a patient who is scheduled to receive therapy because of temporomandibular joint pain. The assistant discovers that the patient has been wearing an inappropriate orthotic in the oral cavity that has caused increased pain and difficulty chewing foods. The physician has ordered treatment of the temporomandibular joint and of the muscles of mastication. Which of the following is not considered a muscle of mastication?

A. Buccinator
B. Platysma
C. Medial pyergoid
D. Temporalis

Question 299.

A PTA is instructing a patient in pre-gait activities who has been fitted with a hip disarticulation prosthesis. To ambulate with the most correct gait pattern, what must be mastered first?

A. Forward weight shift on to the prosthesis
B. Swing-through of the prosthesis
C. Maintain stability while in single limb support on the prosthesis
D. Posterior pelvic tilt to advance the prosthesis

Question 300.

Which of the following is a false statement about below-knee amputations?

A. Gel socket inserts should be left in the prosthesis overnight.
B. The PTA should puncture any blisters that appear on the stump.
C. Areas of skin irritation on the stump can be covered with a dressing and then a nylon sock before donning the prosthesis.
D. When not in use, the prosthesis should be laid on the floor.

Question 301.

A physical therapist and PTA are treating a patient for quadriceps weakness. The assistant knows that if the involved lower extremity is positioned in maximum hip flexion and knee extension, the rectus femoris is in its most ___s___ position, and a contraction from this muscle would be weak. This is often referred to as ___A___ insufficiency.

A. Shortened, active
B. Lengthened, passive
C. Shortened, passive
D. Lengthened, active

Question 302.

A patient is in prone position with his head rotated to the left side. The left upper extremity is placed at his side and fully internally rotated. The left shoulder is then shrugged toward the chin. The PTA then grasps the midshaft of the patient's left forearm. The patient is then instructed to "try to reach your feet using just your left arm." This movement is resisted by the assistant. This test is assessing the strength of what muscle?

A. Upper trapezius
B. Posterior deltoid
C. Latissimus dorsi
D. Triceps brachii

Question 303.

A 67-year-old man with a below-knee amputation presents to an outpatient clinic. His surgical amputation was 3 weeks ago, and his scars are well healed. Which of the following is incorrect information about stump care?

A. Use a light lotion on the stump after bathing each night.
B. Continue with use of a shrinker 12 hours per day.
C. Wash the stump with mild soap and water.
D. Use scar massage techniques.

Question 304.

A physical therapist is evaluating a patient with traumatic injury to the left hand. The therapist asks the patient to place the left hand on the examination table with the palm facing upward. The therapist then holds the second, third, and fifth digits in full extension. The patient is then asked to flex the fourth digit. What movement would be expected by a patient with an uninjured hand, and what muscle or muscles is the therapist restricting?

A. The fourth finger would flex at the distal interphalangeal (DIP) joint only, and the muscle being restricted is the flexor digitorum superficialis.
B. The fourth finger would flex at the proximal interphalangeal (PIP) joint only, and the muscle being restricted is the flexor digitorum profundus.
C. The fourth finger would flex at the DIP joint only, and the muscles being restricted are the lumbricals.
D. The fourth finger would flex at the PIP joint only, and the muscles being restricted are the palmar interosseous.

Question 305.

A clinical instructor is explaining to a PTA student the function of the screw-home mechanism in the knee joint. Part of the therapist's explanation involves teaching the student the movement of the tibia and femur during closed-chain activities. When the knee joint is extended in a closed-chain activity, which of the following statements is true?

A. The femur laterally rotates on the tibia.
B. The femur medially rotates on the tibia.
C. The tibia laterally rotates on the femur.
D. The tibia medially rotates on the femur.

Question 306.

A PTA is treating a patient in order to increase lateral stability of the knee joint. The assistant is using strengthening exercises to strengthen muscle groups that will increase active restraint on the lateral side of the joint. Which of the following offers the least amount of active lateral restraint?

A. Gastrocnemius
B. Popliteus
C. Biceps femoris
D. Iliotibial band

Question 307.

A physical therapist receives an order from the physician to treat a patient using iontophoresis. The order indicates that the purpose of the treatment is to attempt to dissolve a calcium deposit in the area of the Achilles' tendon. The physical therapist then allows a PTA to help treat the patient. When preparing the patient for treatment, the assistant connects the medicated electrode to the negative pole. Which of the following medications is the assistant most likely preparing to administer?

A. Dexamethasone
B. Magnesium sulfate
C. Hydrocortisone
D. Acetic acid

Question 308.

A patient with cardiac arrhythmia is referred to physical therapy services for cardiac rehabilitation. The PTA is aware that the heart receives nerve impulses that begin in the sinoatrial node of the heart and then proceed to which of the following?

A. Atrioventricular node, then to the Purkinje fibers, and then to the bundle branches
B. Purkinje fibers, then to the bundle branches, and then to the atrioventricular node
C. Atrioventricular node, then to the bundle branches, and then to the Purkinje fibers
D. Bundle branches, then to the atrioventricular node, and then to the Purkinje fibers

Question 309.

A PTA is reviewing the chart of a cardiac rehabilitation patient. The assistant notes in the chart that the patient's rhythm strip has revealed that the patient has a resting heart rate of 95 bpm. Which of the following terms best describes this rate?

A. Normal
B. Bradycardia
C. Tachycardia
D. Irregular

Question 310.

A PTA must have a clear understanding of the normal development of the human body to treat effectively and efficiently. Which of the following principles of treatment is incorrect?

A. Early motor activity is influenced primarily by reflexes.
B. Motor control develops from proximal to distal and from head to toe.
C. Increasing motor ability is independent of motor learning.
D. Early motor activity is influenced by spontaneous activity.

Question 311.

A PTA is sent to provide passive ROM to a patient in the intensive care unit. The chart reveals that the patient is suffering from pulmonary edema. The charge nurse informs the assistant that the patient is coughing up a thin, white sputum with a pink tint. Which of the following terms best describes this sputum?

A. Purulent
B. Frothy
C. Mucopurulent
D. Rusty

Question 312.

A PTA is performing chest physical therapy on a patient who is coughing up a significant amount of sputum. The assistant later describes the quality of the sputum in his notes as mucoid. This description tells other personnel which of the following?

A. The sputum is thick.
B. The sputum has a foul odor.
C. The sputum is clear or white in color.
D. The patient has a possible bronchopulmonary infection.

Question 313.

A PTA is scheduled to treat the shoulder of a patient with hepatitis B. The assistant notices no open wounds or abrasions and notices that the patient has good hygiene. The physical therapist has suggested passive ROM to the right shoulder because of adhesive capsulitis. Which of the following precautions is absolutely necessary to prevent the PTA from being infected?

A. The therapist must wear a gown.
B. The therapist must wear a mask.
C. The therapist must wear gloves.
D. None of the above

Question 314.

A supervisor is asked by a hired architect to provide some of the measurements needed to make a new clinic accessible for people who require wheelchairs. Some of the concerns of the architect are the minimal width of the doorways, the steepest slope allowed for the wheelchair ramp at the front entrance, and the minimal height of the bathroom toilet seat. If the supervisor provided measurements based on normal adult-size wheelchair, which of the following lists of measurements would be correct?

A. The minimal doorway width should be 32 inches. The steepest slope allowed is 1:12 (for every 12 feet of horizontal length, the ramp can rise vertically by 1 foot). The minimal toilet seat height is 17 inches.
B. The minimal doorway width should be 32 inches. The steepest slope allowed is 1:14 (for every 14 feet of horizontal length, the ramp can rise vertically by 1 foot). The minimal toilet seat height is 22 inches.
C. The minimal doorway width should be 30 inches. The steepest slope allowed is 1:12 (for every 12 feet of horizontal length, the ramp can rise vertically by 1 foot). The minimal toilet seat height is 24 inches.
D. The minimal doorway width should be 28 inches. The steepest slope allowed is 1:12 (for every 12 feet of horizontal length, the ramp can rise vertically by 1 foot). The minimal toilet seat height is 15 inches.

Question 315.

A patient arrives at an outpatient clinic with an order from a physician for whirlpool and wound care to a lower extremity wound. The PTA decides to set the temperature in the whirlpool at warm. Which of the following settings in degrees Celsius is appropriate?

A. 27.5°C
B. 35.5°C
C. 49°C
D. 60°C

Question 316.

While treating a patient who suffered a complete spinal cord lesion, a PTA notes the following strength grades with manual muscle testing: wrist extensors = 3+/5; elbow extensors = 2+/5; and intrinsic muscles of the hand = 0/5. What is the highest possible level of this lesion?

A. C3
B. C4
C. C5
D. C7

Question 317.

A physical therapist informs a PTA that a patient was recently hospitalized for malfunction of the anterior pituitary gland. Based on this information alone, the assistant knows that there may be problems with the patient's ability to produce which of the following hormones?

A. Adrenocorticotropic hormone, thyroid-stimulating hormone, growth hormone, follicle-stimulating hormone, luteinizing hormone
B. Insulin and glucagon
C. Epinephrine and norepinephrine
D. Cortisol, androgens, and aldosterone

Question 318.

A patient is referred to physical therapy with complaints of sensation loss over the area of the radius of the right upper extremity, extending from the elbow joint distally to the wrist. Therapy sessions are focused on assisting the patient in regaining normal sensation. Which of the following nerves is responsible for sensation in this region?

A. Medial antebrachial cutaneous
B. Lateral antebrachial cutaneous
C. Musculocutaneous
D. Both B and C

Question 319.

A physician ordered a splint for a patient who should keep the thumb of the involved hand in abduction. A new graduate is treating the patient and is confused about the difference between thumb flexion, extension, abduction, and adduction. Which of the following lists is correct?

A. Extension is performed in a plane parallel to the palm of the hand, and abduction is performed in a plane perpendicular to the palm of the hand.
B. Flexion is performed in a plane perpendicular to the palm of the hand, and adduction is performed in a plane parallel to the palm of the hand.
C. Extension is performed in a plane perpendicular to the palm of the hand, and adduction is performed in a plane parallel to the palm of the hand.
D. In referring to positions of the thumb, flexion and adduction are used synonymously, and extension and abduction are used synonymously.

Question 320.

A PTA is treating a patient in the intensive care unit. The therapist notices that the patient is moving his hands and fingers in slow, writhing motions. Which of the following terms best describes this type of movement?

A. Lead-pipe rigidity
B. Ballisms
C. Chorea
D. Athetosis

Question 321.

A patient with chronic back pain is referred to physical therapy for application of a TENS unit. The parameters chosen by the physical therapist are set to provide a noxius stimulus described as an acupuncture type of stimulus. Which of the following lists of parameters produces this type of stimulation?

A. Low intensity, duration of 60 msec, and a frequency of 50 Hz
B. High intensity, duration of 150 msec, and a frequency of 100 Hz
C. Low intensity, duration of 150 msec, and a frequency of 100 Hz
D. High intensity, duration of 150 msec, and a frequency of 2 Hz

Question 322.

A patient with a diagnosis of congestive heart failure is being treated in a cardiac rehabilitation program. This patient suffers from right-sided heart failure. Which of the following is primarily not a result of right-sided heart failure?

A. Jugular vein distension
B. Pulmonary edema
C. Enlarged liver
D. Dependent pitting edema

Question 323.

A physician has ordered a specific type of electrical stimulation that uses a frequency of 2500 Hz with a base frequency at 50 Hz to achieve fused tetany. What type of electrical stimulation has the physician ordered?

A. Iontophoresis
B. TENS
C. Intermittent flow configuration
D. Russian stimulation

Question 324.

A PTA is treating a wound in a patient with the following signs: the right foot has a toe that is gangrenous, the skin on the dorsum of the foot is shiny in appearance, and no calluses are present. The patient has what type of ulcer?

A. Venous insufficiency ulcer
B. Arterial insufficiency ulcer
C. Decubitus ulcer
D. Trophic ulcer

Question 325.

A clinical instructor is explaining to her student how a muscle contracts. The instructor describes the cycle of cross-bridging. She begins by stating that the first step is that the cross-bridges attach to the thin filament. Which of the following occurs next (in the correct order)?

A. The attachment with the actin filament is lost. The cross-bridge moves into position to attach to the thick filament. The cross-bridge moves, causing the thin filament to move.
B. The cross-bridge moves into position to attach to the thick filament. The attachment with the myosin filament is lost. The cross-bridge moves, causing the thin filament to move.
C. The attachment with the myosin filament is lost. The cross-bridge moves, causing the myosin filament to move. The cross-bridge moves into position to attach to a myosin filament.
D. The cross-bridge moves, causing the actin filament to move. The attachment with the thin filament is lost. The cross-bridge moves into position to attach to an actin filament.

Question 326.

Which of the following exercises does not increase strength of the muscles of forceful inspiration?

A. Active cervical flexion exercises
B. Active glenohumeral extension exercises
C. Shoulder shrugs
D. Crunches

Question 327.

A PTA is helping a patient to improve fine motor control of his hands. Which of the following statements is false when comparing methods to improve fine motor control versus improving gross motor control?

A. Use large pieces of material with activities to improve fine motor control and small pieces of material to improve gross motor control.
B. Activities that improve fine motor control usually require less energy expenditure than activities used to improve gross motor control.
C. Activities that improve gross motor control require larger movements than activities used to improve fine motor control.
D. Fine motor activities require a higher degree of accuracy than activities used to improve gross motor skills.

Question 328.

A PTA is treating a 65-year-old man with pneumonia. The patient questions the benefits of the flow incentive spirometer left in the room by the respiratory therapist a few minutes ago. Which of the following is an appropriate response to the patient's question?

A. "It gives visual feedback on lung performance."
B. "It helps you maintain current lung volumes."
C. "You need to ask the respiratory therapist this question."
D. A and B are correct responses

Question 329.

A PTA is speaking to a group of pregnant women about maintaining fitness level during pregnancy. Which of the following statements contains incorrect information?

A. Perform regular exercise routines at least three times per week.
B. Perform at least 15 minutes per day of abdominal exercises in supine position during the second and third trimesters.
C. Increase caloric intake by 300 calories per day.
D. Exercise decreases constipation during pregnancy.

Question 330.

A 45-year-old man with a diagnosis of multiple sclerosis is receiving home health services. The PTA is informed by the supervising therapist that the patient is suffering an acute exacerbation of his condition. Which of the following actions would be appropriate treatment for this patient during this period?

A. Increase the duration of the exercise sessions but decrease the intensity of each exercise performed.
B. Discontinue all exercises.
C. Perform minimal aerobic exercises only.
D. Increase the intensity of the exercises performed but decrease the duration of each session.

Question 331.

Which of the following statements is not a common physiologic change of aging?

A. Blood pressure taken at rest and during exercise increases.
B. Maximal oxygen uptake decreases.
C. Residual volume decreases.
D. Bone mass decreases.

Question 332.

A child with cerebral palsy has been fitted with appropriate positioning equipment to prevent contractures. Which of the following statements is false regarding positioning equipment?

A. Positioning equipment serves to improve ROM.
B. Positioning equipment improves the child's response to the surrounding environment.
C. Positioning equipment provides postural support.
D. Positioning equipment improves body alignment.

Question 333.

A patient complains of pain with right external abdominal oblique contractions secondary to a large hematoma. Which of the following motions would be painful for this patient?

A. Ipsilateral trunk rotation
B. Contralateral trunk rotation
C. Trunk extension
D. Contralateral side bending

Question 334.

A PTA is observing a patient with muscular dystrophy. The patient seems to "waddle" when she walks. She rolls the right hip forward when advancing the right lower extremity and the left hip forward when advancing the left lower extremity. Which of the following gait patterns is the patient demonstrating?

A. Gluteus maximus gait
B. Dystrophic gait
C. Arthrogenic gait
D. Antalgic gait

Question 335.

A PTA is using the technique of proprioceptive neuromuscular facilitation (PNF) to assist a patient in regaining his ability to ambulate. The starting position of the diagonal used by the PTA places the involved lower extremity in maximum hip medial rotation, abduction, and extension. Which of the following PNF diagonals is being used?

A. D2 extension
B. D2 flexion
C. D1 extension
D. D1 flexion

6-23-08

Question 336.

A PTA is treating a patient with complaints of pain on the lateral aspect of the right palm that is increased at night. This patient also has weak pinch strength and noticeable atrophy of the thenar muscles. Which of the following conditions do these signs and symptoms best describe?

A. Rheumatoid arthritis
B. Dupuytren's contracture
C. Carpal tunnel syndrome
D. DeQuervain's disease

Question 337.

A patient with an injured spinal cord has suffered from frequent activation of the sympathetic nervous system caused by an obstructed catheter or any other type of noxious stimulus. The patient and his family have received instruction by the PTA on how to respond when this emergency occurs. The assistant has also educated the family on the effects of activation of the sympathetic nervous system. Which of the following is not a sign or symptom produced by the sympathetic nervous system?

A. Activation of muscles
B. Dilatation of pupils
C. Increased peristalsis
D. Increased blood pressure

Question 338.

A PTA is treating a patient with significant burns over the limbs and upper trunk. Which of the following statements is false about some of the changes initially experienced after the burn?

A. This patient initially experienced an increase in the number of white blood cells.
B. This patient initially experienced an increase in the number of red blood cells.
C. This patient initially experienced an increase in the number of free fatty acids.
D. This patient initially experienced a decrease in fibrinogen.

Question 339.

A patient presents to therapy with poor motor control of the lower extremities. The PTA determines that to work efficiently toward the goal of returning the patient to his prior level of ambulation, he must work in the following order regarding stages of control:

A. Mobility, controlled mobility, stability, skill
B. Stability, controlled stability, mobility, skill
C. Skill, controlled stability, controlled mobility
D. Mobility, stability, controlled mobility, skill

Question 340.

A PTA is asked to treat a patient in the intensive care unit. The patient is comatose but breathing independently. During passive ROM to the right upper extremity, the assistant notices that the patient is breathing unusually. The pattern is an increase in breathing rate and depth followed by brief pauses in breathing. The assistant should notify the appropriate personnel that the patient is exhibiting which of the following patterns?

A. Biot's
B. Cheyne-Stokes
C. Kussmaul's
D. Paroxysmal nocturnal dyspnea

Question 341.

A 4-month-old infant with a diagnosis of congenital talipes equinovarus is scheduled to receive outpatient physical therapy. What would the PTA assistant expect to find during observation of the patient's foot in non–weight-bearing?

A. Pes cavus, adduction of the forefoot, rear foot varus
B. Pes planus, adduction of the forefoot, rear foot varus
C. Pes planus, abduction of the forefoot, rear foot varus
D. Pes cavus, adduction of the forefoot, rear foot valgus

Question 342.

At a team meeting, the respiratory therapist informs the rest of the team that the patient, just admitted to the subacute floor, experienced breathing difficulty in the acute care department. The respiratory therapist describes the breathing problem as a pause before exhaling after a full inspiration. Which of the following is the therapist describing?

A. Apnea
B. Orthopnea
C. Eupnea
D. Apneusis

Question 343.

A supervising therapist informs a physical therapist assistant that a 45-year-old woman has 15° of hind foot valgus and 10° forefoot varus. From this information only, what would the assistant expect to find during treatment of this patient?

A. A foot without deformity
B. Mild pes planus
C. Moderate pes planus
D. Severe pes planus

Question 344.

A PTA is treating a patient in an outpatient facility. The patient has recently been diagnosed with type I insulin-dependent diabetes mellitus. The patient asks the assistant the differences between type I insulin-dependent diabetes mellitus and type II non–insulin-dependent diabetes mellitus. Which of the following statements is true?

A. There is usually some insulin present in the blood in type I and none in type II.
B. Ketoacidosis is a symptom of type II.
C. The age of diagnosis with type I is usually younger than the age of diagnosis with type II.
D. Both conditions can be managed with a strict diet only without taking insulin.

Question 345.

A PTA is treating an infant with the mother present. The assistant suddenly seems to temporarily lose grip of the infant, causing him to be startled and begin to cry. The infant's mother is noticeably upset but is reassured that startling the infant was part of the treatment. Which of the following may the PTA have been assessing?

A. Landau response
B. Symmetric tonic neck reflex
C. Labyrinthine head righting
D. Moro reflex

Question 346.

An infant is being treated by a PTA. The assistant is resisting movement of the right upper extremity and notices involuntary movement of the left upper extremity. Which of the following is displayed by the infant?

A. Landau reaction
B. Startle reflex
C. Moro reflex
D. Associated reaction

Question 347.

A PTA is instructed to test the strength of the splenius cervicis muscles of a 45-year-old man. What motion of the cervical spine should the PTA resist?

A. Extension
B. Flexion
C. Contralateral rotation
D. Contralateral side bending

Question 348.

A patient is referred to physical therapy with a history of temporomandibular joint pain. The PTA notices that the patient is having difficulty closing his mouth against minimal resistance. With this information, which of the following muscles would not be a target for strengthening exercise to correct this deficit?

A. Medial pterygoid muscle
B. Temporalis
C. Masseter
D. Lateral pterygoid muscle

Question 349.

A PTA is in a rehabilitation team meeting about a 58-year-old man with Parkinson's disease. The physician notes that the patient's recent decrease in level of function may be caused by long-term use of a certain drug. The physician plans to take the patient off of the medication for 2 weeks. Which of the following medications is the patient probably taking?

A. Cardizem
B. Cortisone
C. Epinephrine
D. Levodopa

Question 350.

A patient with complaints of foot pain during ambulation is beginning treatment in an outpatient rehabilitation facility. During the evaluation, the medial longitudinal arch is observed in full weight bearing and non–weight bearing. The arch is decreased in both positions. What is the most correct clinical term for this patient's condition?

A. Rigid pes cavus
B. Rigid pes planus
C. Flexible pes cavus
D. Flexible pes planus

Question 351.

A supervising therapist has provided a tennis elbow band to a patient with a diagnosis of lateral epicondylitis. Where should the PTA place the band?

A. Immediately superior to the lateral epicondyle of the humerus
B. Immediately inferior to the lateral epicondyle of the humerus
C. 2 inches below the lateral epicondyle of the humerus
D. Midshaft of the forearm

Question 352.

A 20-year-old man with an anterior cruciate ligament reconstruction with allograft presents to an outpatient physical therapy clinic. The patient's surgery was 5 days ago. The patient is independent in ambulation with crutches. He also currently has 53° of active knee flexion and 67° of passive knee flexion and lacks 10° of full knee extension actively and 5° passively. What is the most significant deficit on which the PTA should focus treatment?

A. Lack of active knee extension
B. Lack of passive knee extension
C. Lack of active knee flexion
D. Lack of passive knee flexion

Question 353.

A supervising therapist evaluates a patient with complaints of elbow pain. The PTA is instructed to perform humeroulnar joint distraction. Which of the following is the correct procedure to perform this task?

A. Place the elbow in full extension. Grasp the forearm just proximal to the wrist and the humerus immediately proximal to the elbow. Apply a traction force on the forearm.
B. Place the patient in prone with the upper extremity hanging from the edge of a treatment table. The shoulder should be in 90° of flexion. Have the patient hold a 10-pound weight in the involved hand.
C. Place the elbow in 130° of flexion. Grasp the mid-shaft of the forearm and the humerus just proximal to the elbow. Instruct the patient to use maximal effort to extend the elbow as the physical therapist assistant resist this motion.
D. Place the patient in supine with the elbow between 70° to 90° flexion. Grasp the forearm immediately distal to the elbow with both hands and apply a distracting force.

Question 354.

A 76-year-old man with complaints of diffuse bilateral lower extremity pain is referred to physical therapy. He is currently ambulating with a standard walker secondary to balance deficits. The referring physician has diagnosed the patient with spinal stenosis. Which of the following exercises would be the most appropriate?

A. Prone press ups
B. Supine single knee to chest
C. Hip bridging
D. Bilateral hip extension while prone over a Swiss ball

Question 355.

A PTA is beginning the treatment of a patient with AIDS. The patient was admitted to the acute floor of the hospital on the previous night after receiving a right total hip replacement. The physician has ordered gait training and a dressing change of the surgical site. Of the following precautions, which is the least necessary?

A. Mask
B. Gloves
C. Handwashing
D. Gown

Question 356.

A patient is being treated with iontophoresis, driving dexamethasone, for inflammation around the lateral epicondyle of the left elbow. The PTA is careful when setting the parameters and with cleaning the site of electrode application to prevent a possible blister. This possibility is not as strong with some other forms of electrical stimulation, but with iontophoresis using a form of _____, precautions must be taken to ensure that the patient does not receive a mild burn or blister during the treatment session.

A. Alternating current
B. Direct current
C. Pulsed current
D. TENS

Question 357.

A PTA is treating a 56-year-old man with a diagnosis of lumbar muscle strain. The referring physician and supervising therapist ruled out neurologic involvement before initiation of treatment. The current plan of care calls for pain relieving modalities and William's flexion exercises. The patient has been performing the lumbar flexion exercise for 2 weeks without adverse reactions. Today he complains of "numbness and tingling" over the lateral left lower extremity. What is the most appropriate course of action by the PTA?

A. Begin McKenzie extension exercises.
B. Contact the referring physician.
C. Advise the patient to discontinue his therapy for 1 week.
D. Contact the supervising therapist.

Question 358.

A PTA is massaging the upper trapezius of a patient. Which one of the techniques involves lifting and kneading of the tissues?

A. Tapotement massage
B. Effleurage massage
C. Petrissage massage
D. Friction massage

Question 359.

A supervising therapist has evaluated a patient with an injury to the acromioclavicular (AC) joint. According to the referring physician and the physical therapist, there is complete rupture of the AC ligament and partial tearing of the coracoacromial ligament. An abnormally prominent distal clavicle can be palpated. What degree of AC joint separation does this patient most likely suffer from?

A. Grade 1 (or first degree)
B. Grade 2 (or second degree)
C. Grade 3 (or third degree)
D. Unable to determine from the information given

Question 360.

A PTA is treating a patient with cystic fibrosis who has just walked 75 feet before experiencing significant breathing difficulties. In an effort to assist the patient in regaining her normal breathing rate, the assistant gives a set of instructions. Which of the following set of instructions is appropriate?

A. "Take a slow, deep breath through pursed lips and exhale slowly through your nose only."
B. "Take small breaths through your nose only and exhale quickly through pursed lips."
C. "Breath in through your nose and exhale slowly through pursed lips."
D. "Breath in through pursed lips and breathe out slowly through pursed lips."

Question 361.

A patient with a spinal cord injury is being treated by physical therapy in an acute rehabilitation setting. The patient has been involved in a motor vehicle accident that resulted in a complete C8 spinal cord lesion. The patient is a 20-year-old man who has expressed concern to the PTA about his future sexual function. Which of the following is the most correct information to convey to this patient?

A. Psychogenic erection is possible, reflexogenic erection is not possible, and ejaculation is possible.
B. Psychogenic erection is not possible, reflexogenic erection is not possible, and ejaculation is not possible.
C. Psychogenic erection is possible, reflexogenic erection is possible, and ejaculation is possible.
D. Psychogenic erection is not possible, reflexogenic erection is possible, and ejaculation is not possible.

Question 362.

A PTA is treating a patient with complaints of low back pain. The patient will soon return to a job that requires heavy lifting of objects from the floor throughout the day. The PTA decides to teach correct lifting techniques. As the patient begins to lift the object from the floor, which of the following would indicate incorrect body mechanics?

A. The posterior spinal ligaments are relaxed.
B. The lumbar spine is in a position of lumbar lordosis.
C. The erector spinea muscles are contracted.
D. There is a posterior pelvic tilt.

Question 363.

A PTA is sent to the intensive care unit to treat a patient (who has been evaluated by a physical therapist) who has suffered a severe recent head injury. While reviewing the patient's chart, the PTA discovers that the patient exhibits decerebrate rigidity. The assistant is likely to find this patient in which of the following positions?

A. The patient will be positioned with all extremities extended and the wrist and fingers flexed.
B. The patient will be positioned with the upper extremities flexed, the lower extremities hyperextended, and the fingers tightly flexed.
C. The patient will be positioned with all the extremities flexed and the wrist and fingers extended.
D. The patient will be positioned with the upper extremities extended, the lower extremities flexed, and the fingers hyperextended.

Question 364.

A PTA places a pen in front of a patient and asks him to pick it up and hold it as he normally would to write. The patient picks the pen up and holds it between the pad of the thumb and the middle and the index fingers. What type of grasp or prehension is the patient using?

A. Palmar prehension
B. Fingertip prehension
C. Lateral prehension
D. Hook grasp

Question 365.

A patient is receiving crutch training 1 day after right knee arthroscopic surgery. The patient's weight-bearing status is toe-touch weight bearing on the right lower extremity. The therapist is instructed to teach the patient how to perform a correct sit to stand transfer. Which of the following is the most correct set of instructions?

A. (1) Slide forward to the edge of the chair; (2) put both the crutches in front of you and hold both grips together with the right hand; (3) press on the left arm rest with the left hand and the grips with the right hand; (4) lean forward; (5) stand up, placing your weight on the left lower extremity; and (6) place one crutch slowly under the left arm, then under the right arm.

B. (1) Slide forward; (2) put one crutch in each hand, holding the grips; (3) place the crutches in a vertical position; (4) press down on the grips; and (5) stand up, placing more weight on the left lower extremity.

C. (1) Slide forward to the edge of the chair; (2) put both the crutches in front of you and hold both grips together with the left hand; (3) press on the right arm rest with the right hand and the grips with the left hand; (4) lean forward; (5) stand up, placing your weight on the left lower extremity; and (6) place one crutch slowly under the right arm, then under the left arm.

D. (1) Place crutches in close proximity; (2) slide forward; (3) place your hands on the arm rests; (4) press down and stand up; (5) place your weight on the left lower extremity; and (6) reach slowly for the crutches and place under the axilla.

Question 366.

A physical therapist is ordered to provide gait training for an 18-year-old girl who received a partial medial meniscectomy of the right knee 1 day earlier. After an evaluation, the PTA is consulted. The patient was independent in ambulation without an assistive device before surgery and has no cognitive deficits. The patient's weight-bearing status is currently partial weight bearing on the involved lower extremity. Which of the following is the most appropriate assistive device and gait pattern?

A. Crutches, three-point gait pattern
B. Standard walker, three-point gait pattern
C. Standard walker, four-point gait pattern
D. Crutches, swing-to-gait pattern

Question 367.

A 37-year-old man fell and struck his left temple area on the corner of a mat table. He begins to bleed profusely but remains conscious and alert. Attempts to stop the blood flow with direct pressure to the area of the injury are unsuccessful. Of the following, which is an additional area to which pressure should be applied to stop bleeding?

A. Left parietal bone 1 inch posterior to the ear
B. Left temporal bone just anterior to the ear
C. Zygomatic arch of the frontal bone
D. Zygomatic arch superior to the mastoid process

Question 368.

A PTA is setting up a portable whirlpool unit in the room of a severely immobile patient. What is the most important task of the assistant before the patient is placed in the whirlpool?

A. Check for a ground fault circuit interruption outlet.
B. Check to make sure the water temperature is below 110°F.
C. Make sure the whirlpool agitator is immersed in the water.
D. Obtain the appropriate assistance to perform a transfer.

Question 369.

Which of the following is the correct method to test for interossei muscular tightness of the hand?

A. Passively flex the proximal interphalangeal (PIP) joints with the metaphalangeal (MP) joints in extension; then passively flex the PIP joints with the MP joints in flexion. Record the difference in PIP joint passive flexion.
B. Passively extend the PIP joints with the MP joints in extension; then passively extend the PIP joints with the MP joints in flexion. Record the difference in PIP joint passive flexion.
C. Passively flex the PIP joints with the MP joints in extension; then passively extend the PIP joints with the MP joints in flexion. Record the difference in PIP joint passive flexion.
D. Passively extend the PIP joints with the MP joints in extension; then passively flex the PIP joints with the MP joints in flexion. Record the difference in PIP joint passive flexion.

Question 370.

A PTA is treating a patient who is participating in cardiac rehabilitation. Because the patient complains of chest pain, the assistant attempts to assess heart sounds with a stethoscope. Which of the following is true about the first sound during auscultation of the heart?

A. The first sound is of the closure of the aortic and pulmonic valves.
B. The first sound is of the closure of the mitral and tricuspid valves.
C. The first sound is of the beginning of ventricular systole.
D. B and C

Question 371.

A PTA is observing a patient with poor motor coordination. The assistant notes that when the patient is standing erect and still, she does not respond appropriately when correcting a backward sway of the body. With the body in a fully erect position, a slight backward sway should be corrected by the body's firing specific muscles in a specific order. Which list is the correct firing order?

A. Bilateral abdominals, bilateral quadriceps, bilateral tibialis anterior
B. Bilateral abdominals, bilateral tibialis anterior, bilateral quadriceps
C. Bilateral tibialis anterior, bilateral abdominals, bilateral quadriceps
D. Bilateral tibialis anterior, bilateral quadriceps, bilateral abdominals

Question 372.

In comparing the use of cold pack and hot pack treatments, which of the following statements is false?

A. Cold packs penetrate more deeply than hot packs.
B. Cold increases the viscosity of fluid, and heat decreases the viscosity of fluid.
C. Cold decreases spasm by decreasing sensitivity to muscle spindles, and heat decreases spasm by decreasing nerve conduction velocity.
D. Cold decreases the rate of oxygen uptake, and heat increases the rate of oxygen uptake.

Question 373.

A patient lacks knee extension passive ROM after receiving a meniscectomy 6 weeks ago. The PTA decides to use joint mobilization techniques to gain knee extension. In which direction should the patellofemoral joint and tibia be mobilized?

A. Patella superiorly; tibia anteriorly
B. Patella inferiorly; tibia anteriorly
C. Patella superiorly; tibia posteriorly
D. Patella inferiorly; tibia posteriorly

Question 374.

A patient with a diagnosis of a Bankhart lesion presents to therapy with a physician's prescription to begin physical therapy. With this information alone, the PTA should know that this patient most likely suffered a/an:

A. Anterior shoulder dislocation
B. Posterior shoulder dislocation
C. Ulnar nerve transposition
D. Median nerve compression

Question 375.

A 60-year-old woman is referred to outpatient physical therapy services for rehabilitation after receiving a left total knee replacement 4 weeks ago. The patient is currently ambulating with a standard walker with a severely antalgic gait pattern. Before the recent surgery, the patient was ambulating independently without an assistive device. Left knee flexion was measured in the initial evaluation and found to be 85° actively and 94° passively. The patient also lacked 10° of full passive extension and 17° of full active extension. Which of the following does the therapist assistant need to address first?

A. Lack of passive left knee flexion
B. Lack of passive left knee extension
C. Lack of active left knee extension
D. Ability to ambulate with a lesser assistive device

Question 376.

A patient is receiving electrical stimulation for muscle strengthening of the left quadriceps. One electrode from one lead wire, 4 × 4 inches in size, is placed on the anterior proximal portion of the left quadriceps. Each of two other electrodes from one lead wire are 2 × 2 inches in size. One of the electrodes is placed on the inferior medial side of the left quadriceps and one on the inferior lateral side of the left quadriceps. This is an example of what type of electrode configuration?

A. Monopolar
B. Bipolar
C. Tripolar
D. Quadripolar

Question 377.

When using electrical stimulation with a unit that plugs into the wall, the PTA must take many different safety precautions. Which of the following precautions would probably not increase safety to the patient and therapist?

A. Never place the unit in close proximity to water pipes while treating a patient.
B. Never use an extension cord when using a plug-in unit.
C. Always adjust the intensity of stimulation during the off portion of the cycle.
D. Both A and C are measures that are not likely to increase safety.

Question 378.

A physical therapist has just finished an initial evaluation of a patient with a diagnosis of impingement of the right rotator cuff. Which of the following exercises should be avoided in early rehabilitation?

A. External rotation strengthening with the upper extremity in 30° of abduction
B. Posterior capsule stretching
C. Serratus anterior wall push-ups
D. Strengthening into 170° of abduction

Question 379.

A PTA is treating a 35-year-old man who has suffered loss of motor control in the right lower extremity caused by peripheral neuropathy. The assistant applies biofeedback electrodes to the right quadricep in an effort to increase control and strength of this muscle group. The biofeedback can help achieve this goal in all of the following ways except:

A. Providing visual input for the patient to know how hard he is contracting the right quadriceps
B. Assisting the patient in recruitment of more motor units in the right quadriceps
C. Providing a measure of torque in the right quadriceps
D. Providing input on the patient's ability and effort in contracting the right quadriceps

Question 380.

A patient is performing straight-leg raises with a 5-pound weight 2 inches proximal to the ankle. During the leg raises, a 5° quadriceps lag is observed. Which of the following actions by the PTA would possibly allow the patient to perform the exercise correctly?

A. Move the weight distally.
B. Move the weight proximally.
C. Decrease the poundage.
D. B and C

Question 381.

Use of short-wave diathermy and microwave diathermy is not contraindicated in which of the following conditions?

A. On a patient who has a pacemaker
B. Over the site of a metal implant
C. On a patient who has hemophilia
D. Using pulsed short wave over an acute injury

Question 382.

A PTA is treating of a 15-year-old boy with chronic anterior compartment syndrome. During the treatment session, the patient complains of increased "numbness and tingling" over the dorsum of the foot. Palpation should occur over what artery and at what location?

A. Dorsalis pedis artery posterior to the medial malleolus
B. Dorsalis pedis artery between the first and second metatarsals
C. Posterior tibial artery posterior to the medial malleolus
D. Posterior tibial artery between the first and second metatarsals

Question 383.

A physician orders a program of closed-chain strengthening exercises for a patient recovering from knee surgery. Which of the following would be contraindicated?

A. Proprioceptive activities on a rocker board
B. Seated isokinetic terminal knee extensions
C. Stair-stepper machines
D. Leg press machines

Question 384.

Which of the following statements is false about cardiovascular response to exercise in trained or sedentary patients?

A. If exercise intensities are equal, the sedentary patient's heart rate increases faster than the trained patient's heart rate.
B. Cardiovascular response to increased workload increases at the same rate for sedentary as it does for trained patients.
C. Trained patients have a larger stroke volume during exercise.
D. Sedentary patients reach anaerobic threshold faster than trained patients, if workloads are equal.

Question 385.

Which of the following circumstances would normally decrease body temperature in a healthy person?

A. Exercising on a treadmill
B. Pregnancy
C. Normal ovulation
D. Reaching age of 65 years or older

Question 386.

A physical therapist has just given the patient a custom wheelchair. The patient has a long-standing history of hamstring contractures resulting in fixation of the knees into 60° of flexion. The patient is also prone to develop decubitus ulcers. The family asks the assistant for advice on preventing decubitus ulcers. Which of the following is incorrect information to convey to this family and patient?

A. Keep the patient's buttocks clean and dry.
B. Make sure that the wheelchair cushion is always in the wheelchair seat.
C. Keep the leg rests of the wheelchair fully elevated.
D. Never transfer using a sliding board from one surface to another.

Question 387.

A PTA is beginning treatment for a 65-year-old woman who has suffered a recent stroke. The occupational therapist informs the PTA that the patient has apraxia. She cannot brush her teeth on command; however, she can point out the toothbrush and verbalize the purpose of the toothbrush. From this information, what sort of apraxia does this patient have? How should the PTA approach treatment?

A. Ideomotor apraxia; the PTA should speak in short, concise sentences.
B. Ideational apraxia; the PTA should always give the patient three-step commands.
C. Ideomotor apraxia; the PTA should always give the patient three-step commands.
D. Ideational apraxia; the PTA should speak in short, concise sentences.

Question 388.

A physical therapist is assessing a 40-year-old man's balance and coordination. The following instructions are given to the patient: "Stand normally, with your eyes open. After 15 seconds, close your eyes and maintain a normal standing posture." Several seconds after closing his eyes, the patient nearly falls. What type of test did the patient fail?

A. Nonequilibrium test
B. Equilibrium test
C. Romberg test
D. B and C

Question 389.

A physician has ordered a physical therapist to treat a patient with chronic low back pain. The order is to "increase gluteal muscle function by decreasing trigger points in the quadratus lumborum." After the evaluation, the assistant is asked to continue treatment for this patient. What is the first technique that should be used by the PTA?

A. Isometric gluteal strengthening
B. Posture program
C. Soft tissue massage
D. Muscle reeducation

Question 390.

A PTA is reviewing the chart of a 15-month-old boy. During the initial evaluation, the infant was placed in the supine position. Pressure was placed on the ball of the infant's foot by the physical therapist, and flexion of the toes was noted. What reflex was the therapist testing?

A. Flexor withdrawal
B. Plantar grasp
C. Proprioceptive placing
D. Spontaneous stepping

Question 391.

Which of the following motor milestones will most likely be delayed with the presence of the reflex described in the above question?

A. Crawling
B. Rolling prone to supine
C. Ambulation
D. Unsupported sitting

Question 392.

A PTA in an outpatient clinic is called into a room to assist an infant who is unconscious and not breathing. The assistant opens the airway of the infant and attempts ventilation. The breaths do not make the chest rise. After the infant's head is repositioned, the breaths still do not cause the chest to move. What should the assistant do next?

A. Give five back blows.
B. Look into the throat for a foreign body.
C. Have someone call 911.
D. Perform a blind finger sweep of the throat.

Question 393.

An acute-care PTA is treating a patient who has suffered a right hip fracture in a recent fall. During the treatment session, the family informs the assistant that the patient suffered a stroke since the physical therapist's evaluation (1 day earlier). The patient's chart has no record of the recent stroke. What should the assistant do first?

A. Immediately call the referring physician and request a magnetic resonance imaging scan.
B. Treat the patient as ordered.
C. Immediately call the referring physician and request a computed tomography scan.
D. Immediately call the supervising physical therapist.

Question 394.

A patient is referred to physical therapy because of hypertension. The physician has ordered relaxation training. The PTA chooses to instruct the patient in the technique of diaphragmatic breathing. Which of the below is the correct set of instructions?

A. Slow the breathing rate to 8 to 12 breaths per minute, increase movement of the upper chest, and decrease movement in the abdominal region.
B. Slow the breathing rate to 12 to 16 breaths per minute, increase movement of the abdominal region, and decrease movement in the upper chest.
C. Slow the breathing rate to 8 to 12 breaths per minute, increase movement of the abdominal region, and decrease movement in the upper chest.
D. Slow the breathing rate to 12 to 16 breaths per minute, increase movement of the upper chest, and decrease movement in the abdominal region.

Question 395.

Which of the following statements is false about treatment with infrared lamps?

A. Near-infrared lamps heat deeper than far-infrared lamps.
B. Infrared lamps heat both sides of an extremity at one time.
C. PTAs can change the intensity of the heat by changing the angle between the beam and the body part being treated.
D. PTAs can change the intensity by placing the lamp closer to the body part being treated.

Question 396.

A PTA is observing a patient's gait. During heel strike to foot flat on the right lower extremity, which of the following does not normally occur?

A. The left side of the pelvis initiates movement in the direction of travel.
B. The right femur medially rotates.
C. The left side of the thorax initiates movement in the direction of travel.
D. The right tibia medially rotates.

Question 397.

A physical therapist chose to work with her patient using fluidotherapy rather than paraffin wax. The patient has lack of ROM and also needs to decrease hypersensitivity. There are no open wounds on the hand to be treated. Which of the following would not be an advantage of using fluidotherapy versus paraffin wax in this scenario?

A. The therapist can manually assist ROM while the patient has his hand in the fluidotherapy and not while in the paraffin wax.
B. The fluidotherapy can be used to assist in desensitation by adjusting air intensity.
C. The fluidotherapy can be provided at the same time as dynamic splinting, and this cannot be done while in paraffin wax.
D. The fingers can be bound with tape while in fluidotherapy and not in paraffin wax to assist gaining finger flexion.

Question 398.

A 50-year-old woman has been receiving treatment in the hospital for increased edema in the right upper extremity. The PTA has treated the patient for the past 3 weeks with an intermittent compression pump equipped with a multicompartment compression sleeve. The patient's average blood pressure is 135/80 mm Hg. The daily sessions are 3 hours in duration. The pump is set at 50, 40, and 30 mm Hg (distal to proximal) for 30 seconds, on and off for 15 seconds. The assistant decides to change the parameters. Of the following changes, which is the most likely to increase the efficiency of treatment?

A. Place the patient in a seated position with the right upper extremity in a dependent position versus supine and elevated.
B. Increase the maximal pressure from 50 to 60 mm Hg.
C. Change the on/off time to 15 seconds on and 45 seconds off.
D. Equalize the sleeve compartments versus having greater pressure distally.

Question 399.

A physician telephones a PTA regarding a patient who is being treated because of right shoulder pain. The patient's active ROM in the involved shoulder is as follows: flexion, 165°; abduction, 125°; and external rotation, 75°. Passive ROM is as follows: flexion, 175°; abduction, 172°; and external rotation, 85°. The physician asks the PTA, "Does this patient have a rotator cuff tear?" What is the most appropriate response by the assistant?

A. Inform the physician that the patient might have a rotator cuff tear and recommend magnetic resonance imaging.
B. Inform the physician that the patient has a rotator cuff tear.
C. Inform the physician that the patient does not have a rotator cuff tear.
D. Allow the physician to speak to the supervising therapist.

Question 400.

A PTA should consider using a form of treatment other than moist heat application on the posterior lumbar region of all of the following patients except:

A. Patient with a history of hemophilia
B. Patient with a history of malignant cancer under the site of heat application
C. Patient with a history of Raynaud's phenomenon
D. Patient with a history of many years of steroid therapy

ANSWERS & EXPLANATIONS

1. The answer is B.

PTAs can assist a patient with dysarthria and dysphagia by (1) providing posture control exercises for the head and trunk, which assist the effectiveness of the respiration muscles in providing air volume for vocalization; (2) providing exercises for the facial musculature, including the lips and tongue, to assist in vocalization; (3) providing effective verbal interaction with the patient; and (4) minimizing any unnecessary stimuli or distractions during physical therapy sessions. Speech therapists are most qualified to work with patients on swallowing techniques for liquids and solids.

2. The answer is D.

The pressure applied by the PTA should be applied as the patient coughs to assist in a forceful exhalation. Placing the heel of 1 hand approximately 1 inch above the umbilicus applies pressure immediately inferior to the diaphragm.

3. The answer is A.

Spondylolisthesis is defined as a superior vertebra slipping too far anteriorly in relation to the vertebra below. The plan of care mentioned in the question contains no contraindications for this patient. Extension (not flexion) exercises should be avoided in patients with a diagnosis of spondylolisthesis because it may exacerbate the problem of vertebral slipping.

4. The answer is D.

D is the correct answer because in the supine position, the abdominal contents are located more superiorly than in the other positions. This places the diaphragm in a more elevated resting position, which allows greater excursion of the diaphragm. The semi-Fowler's position resembles a reclining position, with the knees bent and the upper trunk slightly elevated. The semi-Folwer's position, without an abdominal binder, allows gravity to pull the abdominal contents downward, which does not put the diaphragm in an optimal resting position. However, this is the position of choice for patients with uncompromised innervation of the diaphragm who have chronic respiratory difficulty. The standing and sitting positions present the same problem, but to a greater extent, as semi-Fowler's position.

5. The answer is C.

Correct electrode placement is over the motor points of the involved muscle. The on/off cycle time is usually between 1:3 and 1:5. Fused tetany of a muscle usually occurs between 50–80 hertz, or pps.

6. The answer is B.

Motor input is transmitted via efferent nerves away from the central nervous system (CNS) to the muscles. Visual input is transmitted via the afferent nerves toward the CNS via the afferent nerves.

7. The answer is C.

Because the patient does not have 50% of normal range of motion (ROM) in the gravity eliminated position, 2−/5 is the appropriate grade. Some therapists argue that this is an example of a 1+/5 grade. Sources used in preparation of this examination indicate that there is no grade of 1+/5 with manual muscle testing.

8. The answer is C.

The common peroneal nerve travels over the lateral knee. It is the *least* likely to be injured. The other structures are either within the knee or directly posterior to it.

9. The answer is D.

The five stages of grieving are (in order from first to last) denial, anger, bargaining, depression, and acceptance.

10. The answer is C.

Patients with congestive heart failure often develop an enlarged heart because of the burden of an increased preload and afterload.

11. The answer is B.

An epidural hematoma is blood located between the skull and the outer layer of membrane (dura mater) covering the brain. A subdural hematoma is located between the dura mater and the middle layer covering the brain (the arachnoid membrane). A subarachnoid hematoma is located between the arachnoid membrane and the pia mater (the innermost layer of membrane covering the brain).

12. The answer is B.

In performing contract–relax–contract antagonist in this particular situation, the internal rotators are actively contracted first; the external rotators are contracted next in an effort to increase external ROM. The agonists are the internal rotators (tight muscle group in this situation), and the antagonists are the external rotators. The infraspinatus, teres minor, and supraspinatus assist the external rotators. The subscapularis is an internal rotator. Other larger muscles also participate in rotation, but this question refers only to the rotator cuff muscles.

13. The answer is A.

Any phrase stated by the patient that is relevant information goes into the subjective portion of the note.

14. The answer is D.

To lock the elbow with this type of prosthesis, the patient must extend the humerus and depress the scapula.

15. The answer is D.

A person with spastic quadriplegia presents with talipes equinovarus. This term is synonymous with clubfoot.

16. The answer is B.

Apnea is defined as an absence of breathing. Eupnea is normal breathing. Apneusis is an inspiratory cramp. Orthopnea is difficulty breathing when in a lying position.

17. The answer is D.

This type of orthotic uses tenodesis to achieve opening and closing of the hand. To close the hand, the patient actively extends the wrist. To open the hand, the patient passively flexes the wrist.

18. The answer is A.

Metatarsal pads, metatarsal bars, and rocker bars transfer weight onto the metatarsal shaft. A scaphoid pad is for patients with excessive pronation.

19. The answer is D.

An avulsion fracture is the tearing away of a portion of bone. A greenstick fracture usually occurs in young people and is an incomplete fracture on the convex side of the involved bone. A communited fracture occurs when the bone is broken into pieces. A complicated fracture occurs when a bone has broken and is piercing an internal organ.

20. The answer is D.

A person in a diabetic coma has low blood pressure.

21. The answer is A.

The gluteus medius on the involved side is most likely responsible for this patient's gait deviation, which is commonly referred to as a Trendelenburg gait pattern. This muscle is responsible for holding the pelvis level during single limb support. The right gluteus medius keeps the left side of the pelvis from dropping when in right lower extremity single limb support, and vice versa for the left gluteus medius. A weak gluteus maximus often causes a patient to lean the trunk back when striking the heel on the involved side (or lurching).

22. The answer is B.

The most important therapy for this patient, of the choices mentioned, is joint mobilization. This, combined with passive ROM provided by the therapist, is most likely to assist in regaining shoulder passive ROM for this patient. Most frozen shoulders are limited in the plane of abduction, which is increased by performing an inferior glide.

23. The answer is A.

The second cuneiform of the foot articulates with the first cuneiform, second metatarsal, third cuneiform, and navicular.

24. The answer is C.

This is the loose-packed position of the hip.

25. The answer is B.

Genu valgum is a deformity of the knee that causes an inward bowing of the legs. Genu varus is an outward bowing of the legs. Coxa valgum is a deformity at the hip in which the angle between the axis of the neck of the femur and the shaft of the femur is greater than 135°. In coxa varus, this angle is less than 135°. Pes cavus is an increase in the arch of the foot. Pes planus is a flat foot.

26. The answer is B.

The person should lie down to prevent head injury. Tight clothes are loosened to make sure that nothing is too constricting. Close furniture is moved away for the patient's safety. Nothing should be placed in the patient's mouth because of the danger of obstructing the airway.

27. The answer is B.

A patient with damage to Broca's area is a right hemiplegic. Damage to this area causes difficulty with speaking and sometimes difficulty with writing. Damage to this area usually does not impair the ability to understand written or spoken language.

28. The answer is A.

The ADA allowed structural modifications of federal buildings and protection from discrimination based on disability.

29. The answer is C.

Terminal knee extension exercises are open-chain exercises performed in the range, usually from 30° of full extension, to the full available range of active extension for that particular patient. A patient who has received an anterior cruciate ligament reconstruction usually should avoid open-chain exercises ranging from 0° to 45° of knee flexion (sources vary as to the exact degrees) because these exercises place too much stress on the anterior cruciate ligament, which functions to limit anterior displacement of the tibia on the femur.

30. The answer is C.

The description of this patient's ankle is typical of an acute sprain. The treatment requested is appropriate for this condition.

31. The answer is C.

The capitate should be used as the axis.

32. The answer is D.

Tissue with a high collagen content absorbs more ultrasound. Bone absorbs the most ultrasound.

33. The answer is B.

This patient could just have muscle soreness or a deep vein thrombosis (DVT). A DVT is a life-threatening condition that requires hospitalization and subsequent immobilization because of the danger of the clots dislodging and traveling to the lungs. Some of the signs of a DVT are a positive Homan's sign, increased redness, and increased warmth in the calf region. The patient in this scenario does not fit the ideal because symptoms are most often unilateral and the PTA did not note increased warmth. Not all patients fit the profile exactly. It would be the best decision for the PTA to contact the supervising therapist and other appropriate personnel in this situation.

34. The answer is A.

Torticollis involving the right sternocleidomastoid would cause right lateral cervical flexion and left cervical rotation.

35. The answer is B.

The bone-to-bone end-feel should indicate to the PTA that this may be the maximum amount of elbow extension available passively for this patient, who has a history of arthritis.

36. The answer is B.

This form of spina bifida is associated with direct involvement with the cauda equina. The muscles that are innervated by the cauda equina usually present with flaccid paralysis.

37. The answer is C.

The PTA should wait until they (i.e., the physical therapist and PTA) can both work together with the patient. The family is not qualified to help the assistant during the first attempt at ambulation in this situation.

38. The answer is D.

Hypertension is a risk factor in atherosclerosis.

39. The answer is D.

Dry skin is a sign of a diabetic coma.

40. The answer is A.

Choice A describes an isotonic exercise, choice B is an isometric exercise, and choice C is an isokinetic exercise.

41. The answer is D.

If the foot is outset too much, it is likely to cause the prosthetic knee to bow inward during standing.

42. The answer is A.

Infants accomplish this task between approximately 5 and 10 months of age. The response in choice A would prevent the parent from excessive unnecessary worry. Sources vary widely about the exact month when developmental milestones are reached, but A is the correct answer in this scenario.

43. The answer is B.

With Guillain-Barré syndrome, some permanent damage can result, with loss of sensory or motor function, but most patients make a full recovery in approximately 6 months. This syndrome often starts after a person has had a bout of the flu or a respiratory infection. Therapy is most often vital to complete recovery for these patients.

44. The answer is C.

Choice C describes the symmetric tonic neck reflex. With passive cervical extension, an infant displays upper extremity extension and lower extremity flexion.

45. The answer is A.

The patient will most likely have increased circumduction caused by loss of active dorsiflexion on the involved side. The common peroneal nerve can be compressed if the lower extremities are positioned so that excessive pressure is on the fibular head. This nerve bifurcates into the deep peroneal nerve and the superficial peroneal nerve. The deep peroneal innervates the anterior tibialis, which is responsible for active dorsiflexion.

46. The answer is D.

Choice D describes an expiratory reserve volume, choice A is residual volume, choice B is tidal volume, and choice C is vital capacity.

47. The answer is D.

The tests in choices A, B, and C all assess the integrity of the anterior cruciate ligament. The pivot shift test is performed with the patient in a supine position. The therapist applies a valgus stress with the lower leg internally rotated while passively flexing and extending the knee. The test result is positive if there is instability with this motion. An anterior drawer test is performed by placing the patient in a supine position with the knee in 90°of flexion with the foot being stabilized by the therapist's body. An anterior force is applied to the tibia by the therapist. The therapist is assessing the amount of joint movement and the end feel to determine the integrity of the anterior cruciate ligament. Lachman's test is similar to the anterior drawer test, but the knee is in slight flexion. The McMurray test is used to determine if meniscus damage is present.

48. The answer is C.

Rhythmic stabilization involves a series of isometric contractions of the agonist, then the antagonist.

49. The answer is B.

The spine of the scapula is approximately at T3. The superior angle of the scapula commonly rests at the same level as vertebra T2. The inferior angle of the scapula and xiphoid process represents T7.

50. The answer is D.

The involved upper extremity is in this position because of damage to the C5 and C6 spinal roots.

51. The answer is B.

Boutonnière deformity involves flexion of the proximal interphalangeal joint and extension of the distal interphalangeal joint. Dupuytren's contracture is thickening of the palmar aponeurosis. Claw hand is the result of laceration to the ulnar nerve.

52. The answer is C.

This is called Ober's test, which screens for a tight iliotibial band.

53. The answer is B.

Type II diabetics may be able to control their condition with diet only (depending on the severity of the condition), but type I diabetics need insulin. A person is usually diagnosed with type I diabetes at 25 years of age or younger. A person is usually 40 years old or older when diagnosed with type II diabetes.

54. The answer is C.

A platform walker has a place to rest the forearm, a handgrip, and straps to hold the forearm in place. It is needed for patients who cannot fully use the involved upper extremity for some reason (e.g., fracture, increased pain with weight bearing) that limits functional mobility, preventing use of a standard or rolling walker.

55. The answer is C.

The pelvis is dropping on the right side because the left gluteus medius is weak. The patient may also lean toward the left hip joint to move the center of gravity, making it easier to hold up the right side of the pelvis.

56. The answer is B.

A PTA cannot legally write a discharge summary.

57. The answer is D.

A shuffling gait and difficulty with initiating gait are typical signs of Parkinson's disease.

58. The answer is D.

Graphesthesia is the ability to identify letters, numbers, or designs traced on the skin. Barognosis is the ability to differentiate between different weights. Stereognosis is the ability to differentiate between different sizes and shapes. Texture recognition is the ability to differentiate between textures such as cotton, wool, or silk.

59. The answer is B.

According to the American Heart Association, a person should be determined unresponsive before emergency medical services are activated.

60. The answer is D.

Superficial partial-thickness burns and deep partial-thickness burns are not deep enough to involve the subcutaneous tissue. An electrical burn is complete destruction of the subcutaneous tissue. A full-thickness burn produces moderate subcutaneous tissue damage and little pain.

61. The answer is C.

The axis point is the knee joint. The effort arm is distal to the knee joint at the insertion of the patella tendon. The resistance is at the ankle. A class 2 lever has the resistance arm in the middle, making a longer effort arm than resistance arm. The class 1 lever has an axis in the middle.

62. The answer is D.

Dupuytren's contracture occurs when the palmar aponeurosis becomes thickened, causing increased flexion of the fingers. The main concentration of initial treatment should be on achieving finger extension passively.

63. The answer is A.

The anterior surface of the face and the upper extremity are each considered 4.5% of the body, according to the rule of nines. The anterior trunk is 18%. Each anterior surface of the lower extremities is 9%. The posterior side is the same, respectively. The total groin area is 1%.

64. The answer is C.

The foot drop is caused by a lack of active dorsiflexion. The tibialis anterior is responsible for this motion and is innervated by the deep peroneal nerve.

65. The answer is C.

The acute stage presents with constant burning pain, abnormally fast hair and nail growth, decreased ROM, and increased sensitivity to pain or light touch. The dystrophic phase presents with decreased temperature, cessation of hair and nail growth, pale skin, and muscle atrophy.

66. The answer is A.

The therapist assistant would use a PNF D1 diagonal to encourage the combined movements of hip flexion, adduction, and knee flexion. This diagonal also encourages the combined movements of hip abduction and extension. This is the combination of muscle activity most needed for gait.

67. The answer is C.

This answer is the most appropriate. The PTA cannot guarantee that everything will be okay (answer A) or that the physician is the best (answer B). Answer D is too insensitive.

68. The answer is D.

The right quadriceps is most likely the involved muscle because the patient is spending less time on the right lower extremity because of pain. Step duration is the amount of time between left heel strike and the successive right heel strike. An abnormal amount of time in the stance time of the reference limb is described as a decrease (or increase) of single limb support time. Decreased step length is defined as a short distance between left heel strike and the successive right heel strike.

69. The answer is D.

To assist a patient in developing a tenodesis grip, the PTA should allow the patient's finger flexors to tighten. This grip facilitated by active extension of the wrist, which allows flexion of the fingers because of shortened flexor tendons.

70. The answer is B.

A PTA should never comment on such a serious prognosis before the physician has assessed the laboratory results and consulted with the patient.

71. The answer is D.

The presence of a limp when using one crutch is an indication that the patient is not ready to use just one crutch. Because the patient has also been non–weight bearing for 6 weeks, the next best step for this patient is to gradually increase weight bearing on the left lower extremity. The use of two crutches, at least until the therapist can reassess the patient's gait pattern at the next scheduled session, is necessary to facilitate return of a normal gait pattern. Typically, a patient is not progressed to a lesser assistive device until he or she is able to ambulate with the current assistive device without limping.

72. The answer is D.

The Thomas test helps to determine whether the hip flexors are too tight.

73. The answer is C.

If the assistant is knowledgeable enough about the particular patient in question, it is appropriate to talk to the physician regarding that patient's progress.

74. The answer is D.

Rheumatoid arthritis is a systemic condition, which is why pain is usually symmetrical. Osteoarthritis primarily involves the weight-bearing joints.

75. The answer is C.

A burst fracture causes damage to the spinal cord because bony fragments are pushed posteriorly into the spinal canal. This type of fracture is often accompanied by anterior cord syndrome.

76. The answer is C.

Posting the inservice date on the bulletin board and sending a memo to the department heads is the most effective way to invite everyone interested. Scheduling sessions during lunch often makes it easier for people to attend.

77. The answer is B.

An isotonic exercise can be either eccentric or concentric. All the answers fit into this category with the exception of the wall sits, which are isometric exercises. During an eccentric contraction, lengthening of the muscle takes place. During a concentric contraction, shortening of the muscle takes place. During an isometric contraction, there is no change in muscle length.

78. The answer is D.

One of the main reasons that pelvic floor exercises are beneficial for a pregnant woman is the extra weight of the viscera.

79. The answer is B.

During pregnancy, women normally experience an increase in resting heart rate and a decrease in heart rate during exercise. This change is compared with the heart rate of the particular woman before pregnancy. The other answers are true about pregnancy.

80. The answer is B.

The correct procedure is answer B. Subtracting 1 inch allows correct pressure distribution over the patient's buttocks and thighs.

81. The answer is B.

During an eccentric contraction, there is lengthening of the muscle. During a concentric contraction, there is shortening of the muscle. During an isometric contraction, there is no change in muscle length. During an isokinetic exercise, the machine being used holds the same speed. Because the speed is held constant, the amount of resistance provided by the machine depends on the effort of the person exercising.

82. The answer is C.

The rotator cuff muscles are the supraspinatus, infraspinatus, teres minor, and subscapularis. They form a force couple that holds the humeral head down and into the glenoid fossa. This opposes the superior force of the deltoid muscle.

83. The answer is D.

Riding a stationary bike at 5.5 mph is approximately 3.5 METs. Descending a flight of stairs is approximately 4 to 5 METs. Ironing is approximately 3.5 METs. Ambulating 5 to 6 mph is approximately 8.6 METs.

84. The answer is A.

Statements made by the patient should go in the subjective portion of the note.

85. The answer is B.

To effectively prevent pressure (decubitis) ulcers, patients should be repositioned every 2 hours.

86. The answer is D.

The lateral triangle (composed of the radial head, olecranon process, and lateral epicondyle) is the most likely of the choices to exhibit joint edema. Joint edema is common after surgical procedures.

87. The answer is B.

Rheumatoid arthritis is a systemic condition that commonly involves joints bilaterally. Crepitus can be associated with osteoarthritis or rheumatoid arthritis, but rheumatoid arthritis is most likely in this case.

88. The answer is B.

Choice B best describes the position that causes injury only to the ACL. In most cases, an audible pop indicates a tear of the ACL. Varus or valgus blows to the knee injure the collateral ligaments and possibly the ACL.

89. The answer is C.

The superior pole is in most contact at approximately 90° of knee flexion.

90. The answer is C.

The PTA must stretch the inferior portion of the capsule in an effort to gain abduction of the involved shoulder. This principle is supported by the convex–concave rule.

91. The answer is A.

A defect in the lamina of a vertebra usually occurs first. This defect is called spondylolysis. The vertebra may then slip because of shear forces; this slippage is called spondylolisthesis.

92. The answer is D.

The metacarpophalangeal joint is enclosed in a joint capsule, so it is considered a diarthrodial joint.

93. The answer is A.

Choice A would probably activate increased tone because of the resistance to plantarflexion offered by the spring.

94. The answer is A.

This theory supports the use of a TENS unit for sensory level pain control. The activation of the larger fibers decreases the amount of sensory information traveling to the brain.

95. The answer is C.

This patient has significant limitations actively and passively but because the end-feels are capsular, the patient's first objective should be to improve passive ROM. Of the choices provided, stretching by the PTA would likely be the most effective for this patient in regaining passive ROM.

96. The answer is D.

The PTA should meet with the nephew on his or her own time and review the exercises.

97. The answer is C.

This answer is correct because the most common deformity after a severe burn such as this is hip flexion, hip adduction, knee flexion, and ankle plantarflexion.

98. The answer is B.

The responses of the patient represent the lowest possible score on the Glasgow coma scale. One point is given for each of the listed responses (or lack thereof).

99. The answer is D.

Exercising at the peak time of insulin effect causes hypoglycemia. Insulin causes the liver to decrease sugar production. The body needs increased levels of blood glucose during exercise.

100. The answer is D.

The correct treatment involves debridement of the eschar over the wound. Elase is an enzymatic wound debridement ointment. Lidocaine is an anesthetic. Dexamethasone is a steroid used mainly with iontophoresis. Silvadene is an antimicrobial agent used to prevent infection.

101. The answer is D.

Compression stockings (e.g., Jobst, TED hose) are used with patients who have poor venous return. A patient with chronic arterial disease already has difficulty with getting blood to the lower extremities; there is no need to further inhibit the blood flow.

102. The answer is B.

The fifth lumbar nerve root is impinged because it arises from the spinal column superior to the L4–L5 lumbar disc.

103. The answer is A.

The plantar calcaneonavicular ligament originates on the sustentaculum tali of the calcaneus and inserts on the navicular bone. This ligament, along with the long plantar ligament, plantar aponeurosis, and short plantar ligament, gives support to the longitudinal arch of the foot. Choice A is the most important ligament.

104. The answer is C.

This position places the greatest amount of lateral force on the patella.

105. The answer is A.

The Q angle is the angle between the line of the pull of the quadriceps muscle and a line through the mid patella and tibial tuberosity. An increased Q angle predisposes individuals to lateral subluxation, or dislocation, of the patella.

106. The answer is D.

The supraspinatus tendon is best palpated by placing the patient's involved upper extremity behind the back in full internal rotation.

107. The answer is A.

In the case of a reciprocal click, the initial click is created by the condyle slipping back into the correct position under the disk with opening of the mouth. In this disorder, the condyle is resting posterior to the disk before jaw opening. With closing, the click is caused by the condyle's slipping away from the disk.

108. The answer is A.

The intervertebral disk has the greatest amount of fluid at the time of birth. The fluid content decreases as people age.

109. The answer is D.

The latissimus dorsi does not participate in external rotation but does contribute in shoulder internal rotation, adduction, and extension.

110. The answer is C.

There are seven cervical vertebrae and eight cervical spinal nerves, thus C8 spinal nerve exits above T1 vertebra.

111. The answer is D.

Dexamethasone is a common antiinflammatory drug driven with the negative electrode. Lidocaine is a commonly used analgesic driven with the positive electrode.

112. The answer is C.

It is possible to use ultrasound on an acute injury, with edema and warmth, when using the machine in the pulse mode with a low duty cycle. The other choices are contraindicated because of the heat generated.

113. The answer is D.

Choices A and C provide the most medial/lateral ankle support. A posterior leaf-spring AFO only provides assistance with dorsiflexion.

114. The answer is A.

The first course of action is to apply direct pressure to the bleeding site in an effort to allow the blood to clot. Use of a tourniquet is no longer recommended unless the bleeding is severe, direct pressure has failed, and the injured person cannot reach emergency medical services in a reasonable amount of time.

115. The answer is B.

A rating of 9 corresponds with "very light." A rating of 7 is "very, very light." A rating of 13 is "somewhat hard." A rating of 15 is "hard." A rating of 17 is "very hard." A rating of 19 is "very, very hard."

116. The answer is C.

When determining the axis and the plane of motion, the body must be visualized in the anatomical plane. The following terms can be used synonomously: coronal and frontal plane, transverse and horizontal plane, vertical and longitudinal axis. Any plane that divides the body into equal parts can be referred to as a cardinal plane. The different axes are vertical axis, (a line through the joint superiorly to inferiorly), sagittal axis (a line through the joint anteriorly to posteriorly) and frontal axis (a line through the joint medially to laterally).

117. The answer is C.

The metacarpophalangeal joint moves in two planes: flexion/extension, and adduction/abduction.

118. The answer is B.

A decreased TV is caused by a restrictive lung dysfunction. An increased TV is caused by an obstructive lung dysfunction.

119. The answer is D.

The fastest settings are appropriate for isokinetic testing. A pitcher's throwing motion is quite fast. It is better to treat with the isokinetic speed as close as possible to the speed of the tested activity.

120. The answer is A.

Claudication is a lack of blood flow. This test is performed by having the patient walk on a treadmill and recording how long the patient can walk before the onset of claudication. Homan's sign is a test performed to see whether a patient may have a deep vein thrombosis. The percussion test is designed to assess the integrity of the great sapheneous vein.

121. The answer is B.

D2 flexion patterns support upper trunk extension, which is important for patients with Parkinson's disease, who tend to develop excessive kyphosis.

122. The answer is A.

Abdominal muscles attach to the lower border of the ribs and the superior surface of the pelvis. Strong abdominal muscles prevent excessive anterior rotation of the pelvis during gait.

123. The answer is B.

The patient probably has a low left shoulder, prominent right scapula, and high left hip.

124. The answer is B.

Rhonchi is commonly described as snoring sounds that can be heard when listening to the breathe sounds of a patient who suffers from chronic bronchitis, during inspiration or expiration. Rales and crackles are sounds during auscultation that commonly occur during the inspiratory phase of breathing and are caused when air opens fluid-filled alveoli. Wheezes are abnormal breath sounds that are produced when air enters tracheobroncial airway passages that are abnormally narrow.

125. The answer is A.

Only the edges of the adult meniscus are vascularized by the capillaries from the synovial membrane and joint capsule.

126. The answer is D.

Policies can be viewed as the rules, and procedures are the ways in which the rules are carried out.

127. The answer is B.

The patient should exercise the right hip abductor muscle group without weight first to quickly obtain full active ROM. The patient should obtain full active ROM with gravity as resistance first before adding ankle weights.

128. The answer is C.

The crutches should not touch the axilla during fitting, with or without axillary pads. The patient should also be encouraged not to place weight on the axilla during ambulation because it could cause injury to the brachial plexus.

129. The answer is D.

The subscapularis, teres minor, and infraspinatus muscles oppose the superior pull of the deltoid muscle. The supraspinatus does not oppose the pull of the deltoid but is important because (along with the other cuff muscles) it provides a compression force to the glenohumeral joint.

130. The answer is B.

A fibers are the largest in diameter and conduct faster than C fibers.

131. The answer is A.

Controlled coughing is similar to huffing, but in huffing, the patient closes the mouth before forcefully exhaling. A splinted cough occurs when a pillow is held up to the area of an incision site during a controlled cough. Huffing is used when controlled coughing or splinting is too strenuous for the patient. Pacing is the method of breaking down an activity into several parts to prevent dyspnea.

132. The answer is D.

A belt that is angled at 90° with the sitting surface limits the patient's involuntary efforts to hyperextend the trunk because of increased tone. This angle also allows the patient to actively tilt the pelvis anteriorly, which is a functional movement that does not need to be restricted.

133. The answer is D.

For many cardiac patients, performing isometric exercises places too much load on the left ventrical of the heart.

134. The answer is D.

This position places the least amount of stress on the lumbar spine in the sitting position.

135. The answer is B.

The area of contact between the humerus and the glenoid fossa is maximal in this position.

136. The answer is D.

This answer is correct because patients need a written home program with diagrams and instructions. One-on-one teaching is also necessary to ensure that patients understand the program. Bringing in another family member is also definitely advisable to assist patients with the program at home.

137. The answer is D.

Answer A is incorrect because any way to solve this problem without denying needed therapy needs to be explored first. Answer B is incorrect because the PTA may be donating a considerable amount of time. This solution is not profitable for the assistant and is likely to cause an uncomfortable working atmosphere. Answer C is incorrect because the matter may be resolved without quitting. Answer D is correct because the immediate supervisor may be able to help the assistant in coming to an agreement between the assistant and the employer.

138. The answer is B.

Answer B is the most empathetic response. It also lets the patient know that the therapists will make an effort to prevent the problem from recurring.

139. The answer is D.

The answer is none of the above because the sacroiliac joint of an 87-year-old woman is fused.

140. The answer is A.

The lowest point in the gait cycle occurs when both lower extremities are in contact with the ground (double support).

141. The answer is D.

Placing a block under the right foot when this patient is in a vertical position would allow non–weight bearing on the involved left lower extremity.

142. The answer is C.

This scenario describes a central cord lesion. It is common in the geriatric population after cervical extension injuries (e.g., whiplash).

143. The answer is B.

A socket that is too large may cause the prosthetic limb to "drop" during ambulation.

144. The answer is C.

Swan-neck deformity involves hyperextension of the proximal interphalangeal joint and flexion of the distal interphalangeal joint. Boutonnière deformity involves flexion of the proximal interphalangeal joint and extension of the distal interphalangeal joint.

145. The answer is B.

The setting of 55° is the most appropriate of the choices offered. A setting of 65° or higher would likely not be tolerated by the patient for an entire night because it took a 30-minute session of maximum effort to achieve 65° of knee flexion.

146. The answer is C.

In static standing, the line of gravity is posterior to the hip joint. The body first relies on the anterior pelvic ligaments and the hip joint capsule. The iliopsoas may be recruited at times, but the anterior ligaments are used first to keep the trunk from extending in static stance.

147. The answer is B.

Choice B is the correct answer. Choice A is a posterior pelvic tilt.

148. The answer is A.

Choice A describes rheumatoid arthritis, a systemic condition. All of the other choices are signs and symptoms of OA. Sometimes OA can involve symmetrical joints, but it is not systemic.

149. The answer is A.

Isometric exercises in the shortest range of the extensor muscle are used to begin strengthening. In contrast, weak flexor muscles should be strengthened in the middle-to-lengthened range because they most often work near their end range.

150. The answer is A.

Ortolani's test is used to detect a congenitally dislocated hip in infants. Choices B and C are common meniscus damage tests for the knee. Choice D is performed by placing the infant in a supine position with the hip at 90° of flexion and slight abduction and the knee flexed to 90°. The examiner then moves the infant's hip anterior and posterior in an effort to detect abnormal joint mobility.

151. The answer is A.

Choice A is the correct gait sequence for ascending stairs in the given scenario. A caregiver should stand below the patient because the patient is most likely to fall *down* the stairs. This same rule holds true for descending stairs.

152. The answer is A.

A patient can obtain his or her medical records simply by signing a release form and paying a fee if required. Charts and records should never be given or faxed to an attorney unless the patient has signed a release form.

153. The answer is D.

Increased spasticity of the left gastrocnemius causes an increase in plantarflexion. Hypotonicity of the tibialis anterior causes a foot drop caused by an inability to dorsiflex actively. A leg length discrepancy is a possibility in any patient, regardless of the diagnosis. The least likely cause of this deficit is a hypertonic left quadriceps, which most likely would cause an increase in dorsiflexion on the involved side in an effort to decrease the functional leg length.

154. The answer is C.

Although sources vary widely, a child can usually sit unsupported between age 4 and 8 months. Answers A and B are incorrect. Answer D would possibly cause the parent to worry prematurely.

155. The answer is A.

Choice A is approximately 6 to 7 METs. Choice B is approximately 4.6 METs. Choice C is approximately 2 METs. Choice D is approximately 3 to 5 METs.

156. The answer is B.

The obturator nerve innervates the adductor brevis, adductor longus, adductor magnus, oburator externus, and gracilis muscles. Choice A has no motor function. Choice C innervates the sartorius, pectineus, iliacus, and quadriceps femoris. The ilioinguinal nerve innervates the obliquus internus abdominis and transversus abdominis.

157. The answer is B.

A lesion at choice A would cause bitemporal heteronymous hemianopsia. A lesion at choice C would cause left eye blindness, and a lesion at D would cause right eye blindness.

158. The answer is A.

Local vasoconstriction is the first response. Nerve conduction velocity decreases after approximately 5 minutes of ice application.

159. The answer is A.

Separation of the intervertebral foramen is best accomplished with the spine in flexion. The positioning of the spine in a neutral position would separate the disk space.

160. The answer is B.

Bifid spinous processes (i.e., spinous processes that are split) are found only in the cervical spine.

161. The answer is D.

An ulnar nerve compromised hand presents as a "claw" hand after a prolonged amount of time because of atrophy of the interossei. The extensor digitorum takes over and pulls the MCP joints in hyperextension.

162. The answer is C.

The age-adjusted maximum heart rate is calculated by subtracting a person's age from 220. Sometimes a patient may have to exercise in a range of 60% to 80% of their maximal heart rate for safety reasons. This is done simply by multiplying 0.6 by the age adjusted maximum heart rate for the bottom number of the range and multiplying by 0.8 for the top number of the range.

163. The answer is A.

The ratings are I—no response; II—generalized response; III—localized responses; IV—confused agitated; V—confused inappropriate; VI—confused appropriate; VII—automatic appropriate; and VIII—purposeful and appropriate.

164. The answer is B.

The cane should be lowered first, followed by the involved lower extremity. As the patient's balance and coordination improve, the cane and involved lower extremity may be lowered first and together. Also, even though the cane is commonly used with the upper extremity on the opposite side of the involved lower extremity, a handrail should be used when possible.

165. The answer is A.

A blood sugar value of 300 mg/dL is a contraindicated level for therapeutic exercise.

166. The answer is B.

The patient can be successfully treated by using universal precautions. The patient should be treated in a relatively isolated area because of his weakened immune system. The diagnosis of AIDS with Kaposi's sarcoma is an indication that the patient's immune system is weak. Gloves should be used if the patient's sarcomas are open; otherwise, handwashing before and after patient contact is appropriate.

167. The answer is C.

The PTA should notify the supervising therapist. The mistake should be documented and the patient informed. The supervising therapist can determine the need for a consultation with a physician.

168. The answer is D.

The standard walker is the most stable, and the straight cane is the least stable of the devices listed. The standard walker requires the least coordination, and the forearm crutches require the most coordination of the devices listed.

169. The answer is A.

Choice A is the correct postural drainage. Choice B is drained by resting on the right, 1/4 turn to the back, and foot of the bed elevated 12 to 16 inches. Choices C and D are drained with the patient in a long sitting position or leaning forward over a pillow in a sitting position.

170. The answer is D.

The patient should lean forward when assuming the standing position. This assists in placing the center of gravity over the base of support.

171. The answer is B.

The diastolic pressure is represented by the bottom number, and the systolic pressure is represented by the top number, when recording a person's blood pressure. A therapist can usually expect an increase in the diastolic pressure, but exercise should definitely be stopped if the diastolic pressure exceeds 130 mm Hg. Some sources recommend termination of exercise when diastolic pressure exceeds 115 mm Hg.

172. The answer is B.

The patient is experiencing autonomic dysreflexia. The correct actions are to find the probable cause of the noxious stimulus and to lower the patient's blood pressure by inducing orthostatic hypotension. Patients with spinal cord injury above the level of T6 can experience this problem.

173. The answer is C.

The lateral collateral ligament of the knee is best palpated with the patient in the sitting position. The patient then places the foot of the involved lower extremity on the knee of the uninvolved lower extremity. This maneuver places the involved knee in 90° of flexion and the hip in external rotation.

174. The answer is B.

Choice B describes fast-twitch muscle fibers. Choice A describes slow-twitch fibers. Choices C and D are incorrect answers.

175. The answer is C.

Obstructed lymph vessels will not allow the compression provided by the pump to adequately move the fluid. Compression over an infected area may spread the bacteria to other sites. Also, a patient must have kidneys that are functioning well enough to excrete additional fluid caused by the compression pump.

176. The answer is C.

A PTA can do all of the listed options except change the frequency or duration as prescribed by a therapist or physician. Choice B allows the PTA to work within the protocol established by the physical therapist.

177. The answer is A.

Information regarding the patient's lifestyle or home situation, provided by a caregiver, should be found in the subjective portion of the initial assessment.

178. The answer is C.

Muscle viscosity increases with cold application, thus slowing movement of the involved area.

179. The answer is C.

A suberythemal dose of ultraviolet treatment is not enough to cause reddening of the skin. A minimal erythemal dose leads to slight itching and reddening. A third-degree erythemal dose is a more severe reaction with blister and edema formation.

180. The answer is C.

Leaning the trunk over the involved hip decreases joint reaction force and strain on the hip abductors. Together, these factors decrease pain in the involved hip.

181. The answer is B.

Grade I is a small oscillating movement at the beginning of range, grade III is a large movement up to the end of available range, and grade IV is a small movement at the end of available range.

182. The answer is A.

The danger in using a hot tub for a person with multiple sclerosis is that it may cause extreme fatigue. There is no need to avoid the other activities listed.

183. The answer is D.

Patellofemoral joint reaction forces increase as the angle of knee flexion and quadriceps muscle activity increase. Choice D involves the greatest knee flexion angle and quadriceps activity.

184. The answer is D.

The supervising therapist will most likely perform another evaluation because of the change in the patient's status. A PTA should not independently begin treatment on a diagnosis that was not included in the initial plan of care.

185. The answer is C.

Parkinson's disease and dementia are disorders that involve the brain. Myasthenia gravis is a problem with acetylcholine receptors at the neuromuscular junction.

186. The answer is B.

Answers A and C are incorrect because rheumatoid arthritis is a contraindication for continuous or intermittent traction. Answer D is incorrect for the above reason as well as the fact that a 110-pound setting is too great for a 147-pound patient.

187. The answer is B.

The gastrocnemius prevents excessive dorsiflexion, and the hamstrings prevent excessive hip flexion.

188. The answer is B.

The iliofemoral ligament is the strongest ligament in the hip that prevents extension. It is the ligament most likely to be compromised in this scenario.

189. The answer is C.

The pitcher is moving into D2 extension with the throwing motion. He is strengthening the muscles involved in shoulder internal rotation, adduction, and forearm pronation.

190. The answer is A.

The motions of plantarflexion and inversion are the mechanism of injury for anterior talofibular ligament ankle sprains, so they should be avoided in early rehabilitation.

191. The answer is C.

Standing with lumbar flexion causes the most intradiscal pressure of the choices given. Increased intradiscal pressure forces the nucleus pulposus to move posteriorly.

192. The answer is A.

A PTA's main responsibility with this patient is to maintain ROM. Fluid retention is an important concern for other medical staff members. Choices C and D will be addressed later in the patient's course of therapy.

193. The answer is A.

The briefcase should be carried in the right hand. Carrying the briefcase in the left hand would increase the amount of force that the right gluteus medius would have to exert to maintain a stable pelvis during gait.

194. The answer is D.

Plyometric exercises are high velocity, demanding exercises used in the latter stages of rehabilitation. Plyometrics involve an eccentric load to a muscle followed by a quick concentric contraction.

195. The answer is C.

A PTA can use ultrasound with all of the other choices. Performing an ultrasound over a cemented metal implant is also a contraindication. However, with any ultrasound technique, treatment should be stopped if the patient experiences pain.

196. The answer is D.

Choices A, B, and C would increase the functional length of the right lower extremity and possibly cause circumduction during gait. Choice D would not change the functional leg length.

197. The answer A.

Salter-Harris fractures involve the epiphyseal plate of a bone.

198. The answer is B.

Direct current is shown to have the greatest benefit in wound healing. Monophasic pulsed current has also been shown to have wound-healing benefits.

199. The answer is C.

Ultrasound is contraindicated in this patient because of the possibility of damage to the epiphyseal growth plate. All other treatments suggested are normally performed with this diagnosis.

200. The answer is C.

Spina bifida occulta is a benign disorder. It presents with no decrease in function. There is no protrusion of the spinal cord or its associated structures, as in choices A and B.

201. The answer is B.

The superior angle of the scapula commonly rests at the same level as vertebra T2. The spine of the scapula is approximately at T3. The inferior angle of the scapula and xiphoid process represents T7.

202. The answer is D.

The long toe extensors are innervated by the spinal cord segment L5. The iliopsoas is innervated by L2. The quadriceps are innervated by L3, and the tibialis anterior is innervated by L4.

203. The answer is A.

This deviation is commonly referred to as a lateral heel whip. Excessive internal rotation of the prosthetic knee is one of the causes of this deviation. Excessive external rotation of the knee causes a medial heel whip.

204. The answer is A.

Ultrasound at 3.0 MHz should be used to treat structures that are up to 2 cm below the surface of the skin. Structures more than 2 cm below the surface of the skin best respond to ultrasound at 1.0 MHz.

205. The answer is A.

A heel that is too stiff causes excessive knee flexion. Choices B and C cause excessive knee extension during this stage of the gait cycle.

206. The answer is C.

Geriatric patients have a longer period of double support in an attempt to maintain balance. They also have a shorter step and stride length.

207. The answer is A.

The hamstrings bring the knee to approximately 60° of flexion during acceleration. The hip flexors, ankle dorsiflexors, and toe extensors are also active.

208. The answer is B.

Viscosity is the friction of fluids. Buoyancy is the property that pushes up on the part immersed with a pressure that is equal to the weight of the amount of water displaced by that part. Relative density states that if the specific gravity of an object is less than 1, it will float; if it is greater than 1, it will sink. Hydrostatic pressure is the property of water that places pressure equally on the immersed part.

209. The answer is A.

The tibialis anterior, extensor digitorum longus, and extensor hallucis longus muscles contract concentrically to achieve a neutral ankle position before initial contact.

210. The answer is D.

Choice D is the length of stride during one gait cycle. Choice A describes a decreased step length, choice B describes a decrease in step duration, and choice C describes a decrease in single limb support time.

211. The answer is B.

To maintain balance, the lumbar spine must laterally flex toward the supporting lower extremity during single limb support.

212. The answer is D.

A patient with hammer toes exhibits hyperextension of the distal interphalangeal joints and metatarsophalangeal joints and flexion of the proximal interphalangeal joints.

213. The answer is D.

A patient with severe knee flexion contractures has a line of gravity that is anterior to the hip, posterior to the knee, and anterior to the ankle. This causes a flexion moment at the hip, knee, and ankle.

214. The answer is D.

In advanced peripheral arterial disease, the patient cannot dissipate the heat associated with continuous ultrasound or hot packs. Application of cold packs may increase vasoconstriction in an area already lacking proper blood flow.

215. The answer is D.

The Golgi tendon organs monitor tension at the musculotendinous junction. Ruffini endings are located in the joint capsule, ligaments, and deep layers of the dermis. Meissner's corpuscles are located in the dermis. Merkel's disks are located below the epidermis.

216. The answer is C.

Tools with small handles require more grip strength. Tasks below shoulder height reduce the risk of impingement, and more force can be applied to tasks if they are kept below elbow height.

217. The answer is B.

The weight should be decreased until the patient can perform a straight leg raise without a quadriceps lag.

218. The answer is C.

The wrists should be in a neutral position when the fingers are on the middle row of the keyboard.

219. The answer is A.

Lateral step-ups are probably too difficult for a patient who received an anterior ligament reconstruction with a patella tendon autograft 2 weeks ago.

220. The answer is A.

When the hindfoot is pronated, the forefoot (transverse tarsal joints) can compensate for uneven terrain. If the hindfoot is supinated, the forefoot is also likely to supinate and possibly cause damage to the lateral ankle ligaments.

221. The answer is D.

The muscle spindles are responsible for the stretch reflex. When a muscle is stretched too quickly, the muscle spindles cause the muscle to contract and shorten (which is the stretch reflex). The Golgi tendon organs are responsible for the inverse stretch reflex. They are located in the junction between the muscle and tendon and detect changes in tension. When a tendon is stretched too quickly, the Golgi tendon organs cause the muscle to relax.

222. The answer is D.

Because of the length of the time since the surgical procedure, the patient may have adhesive capsulitis. The capsule should continue to be stretched to increase ROM. The patient should visit the physician if the ROM deficits continue.

223. The answer is B.

Tarsal tunnel syndrome is caused by compression of the posterior tibial nerve as it travels through the tarsal tunnel. The tarsal tunnel is formed by the medial malleolus, medial collateral ligament, talus, and calcaneus.

224. The answer is D.

With a separation of this size, the PTA should use gentle abdominal strengthening while binding the abdominal region.

225. The answer is D.

This is the most stable position of the hip, which allows more normal growth.

226. The answer is B.

The extensor carpi ulnaris is frequently subluxed after rupture of the triangular fibrocartilage complex. Subluxation leads to many mechanical changes in the wrist that are common in patients with rheumatoid arthritis.

227. The answer is B.

The greater trochanter is considered the axis of rotation for the hip in this position.

228. The answer is C.

Swan neck deformity involves hyperextension of the proximal interphalangeal (PIP) joint and flexion of the distal interphalangeal (DIP) joint. Splinting to avoid this deformity is the treatment of choice. Boutonnière deformity involves flexion of the PIP joint and DIP joint hyperextension. Dupuytren's contracture is contracture of the palmar aponeurosis. Claw hand is the result of laceration of the ulnar nerve.

229. The answer is C.

The lateral aspect of the radial styloid process is considered the axis of carpometacarpal abduction and adduction.

230. The answer is D.

Hip flexion exercises would increase anterior pelvic tilt. None of the other choices would exacerbate forward flexed posture.

231. The answer is A.

A tight iliopsoas bilaterally will increase anterior pelvic tilt. The spine will most likely compensate for this with increased lumbar lordosis and increased thoracic kyphosis.

232. The answer is B.

A grade of 5/5 would require the patient's arms to be folded behind the head. A grade of 3/5 should be given if the inferior angles of the scapulae only clear the treatment table if the arms are outstretched.

233. The answer is D.

The primary hip abductors are the gluteus medius and minimus. They are innervated by the superior gluteal nerve, which arises from L4-S1 within the lumbosacral plexus.

234. The answer is B.

The last position (3 inches) of the grip strength dynamometer isolates the extrinsic muscles of the hand (i.e., the muscles located in the forearm). The closer positions test the intrinsic muscles.

235. The answer is D.

The hip strategy is used to compensate for large movements in the center of mass, and the ankle strategy is used to compensate for small movements.

236. The answer is A.

Initially, level of consciousness should be determined. If the patient is unconscious, then cardiopulmonary resuscitation (airway, breathing, and circulation) should begin.

237. The answer is D.

These values are consistent with the normal physiologic response to exercise. Exercise should be terminated if systolic BP is above 240 mm Hg or diastolic BP is above 110 mm Hg. This patient has an age-predicted maximum heart rate of 145 bpm, so 100 bpm is a reasonable exercising HR.

238. The answer is C.

The triangular fibrocartilage complex is made up of the dorsal radioulnar ligament, ulnar collateral ligament, ulnar articular cartilage, volar radioulnar ligament, ulnocarpal meniscus, and sheath of the extensor carpi ulnaris.

239. The answer is A.

Tennis elbow results from overuse of the wrist extensors. The shoulder's external rotators should be used to power a backhand tennis stroke.

240. The answer is B.

The extensor carpi radialis brevis absorbs most of the stress placed on the involved upper extremity in the position of wrist flexion, ulnar deviation, forearm pronation, and elbow extension (as with a backhand swing in tennis).

241. The answer is D.

An infected wound usually has an odor, and presents with yellowish-green drainage. *Macerated* refers to an excessively moist wound, and *indurated* refers to a dry or hardened wound.

242. The answer is A.

A valgus stress is most likely to injure any medial elbow structures, such as the ulnar nerve. The structures on the lateral side are likely to be injured with a varus stress. Choice C originates on the lateral supracondylar ridge.

243. The answer is D.

An allograft is from another human. Xenograft and heterodermic grafts are synonomous terms used to describe a graft taken from another species. An autograft is taken from the person's own body.

244. The answer is D.

The treatment techniques should be performed in the order of mobility, stability, controlled mobility, and skill.

245. The answer is D.

When an exaggerated symmetrical tonic labyrinthine reflex is present, supine positioning increases extensor tone, and prone positioning increases flexor tone. Sidelying also provides an opportunity for the PTA to stimulate flexion.

246. The answer is D.

Decubitus ulcers are more likely to form over bony prominences. Constant pressure over these areas causes ischemia and eventually tissue death.

247. The answer is A.

A donut pad may produce an area of ischemia around the wound.

248. The answer is B.

The patient has an extension lag, which may be caused by any source that has inhibited the quadriceps and results in an inability to fully extend the knee actively.

249. The answer is A.

This is the primary function of the anterior inferior tibiofibular ligament.

250. The answer is D.

The posterior cruciate ligament becomes tight in full knee extension. This assists the tibia in external rotation, which is needed for the screw-home mechanism with open-chain activities.

251. The answer is B.

Plantarflexors have to contract in quiet standing. Other muscles are recruited with movement of the center of gravity.

252. The answer is C.

At 1 to 2 weeks after surgery, the patient has an inflamed knee, and no functional testing can take place. Six weeks is an appropriate amount of time to allow inflammation to decrease enough for functional testing. Patients who have received a partial meniscectomy do not require as much healing time as patients who have received a meniscus repair.

253. The answer is B.

A correct transfer requires the hands anterior to the hips in order to facilitate a forward trunk lean. An upper trunk twist to the right moves the buttock to the left.

254. The answer is D.

If the supervising therapist has determined that progress will no longer be made, the patient should be discharged. The physical therapist can contact the referring physician or social services if necessary. Choice C is incorrect because it is not an empathetic response.

255. The answer is C.

Alzheimer's patients require consistent sequencing of events. Three- to four-step commands and crowded rooms might confuse the patient.

256. The answer is C.

The fingers should be wrapped separately to keep the skin from adhering. Also, wrapping the fingers individually would allow the patient to perform ROM exercises. Anchoring the bandage over the dorsum of the hand will ensure good coverage of the wound and keep the bandage from slipping.

257. The answer is D.

To avoid contamination, gloves should be the last article donned. If gloves are used first, they will become contaminated by touching the other articles of protection.

258. The answer is B.

The patient is prone to excessive external rotation when attempting to extend the involved hip because the gluteus minimus counteracts the lateral rotational force created by the gluteus maximus.

259. The answer is A.

If the patient is pushed way from the PTA, then there is a chance that the patient could roll off the bed. The PTA's body can stop this roll if the patient is rolled toward him. Placement of the left ankle over the right ankle helps facilitate a roll to the right and vice versa for a roll to the left.

260. The answer is B.

The anterior cruciate ligament is located within the articular cavity but outside the synovial lining. The anterior and posterior cruciate ligaments have their own synovial lining.

261. The answer is C.

The handgrips are fitted in the same manner as a cane or walker. The cuffs should be inferior to the elbow.

262. The answer is C.

A sidelying position with a pillow between the knees places less stress on the lumbar area than prone positioning. Supine positioning without a pillow under the knees places too much stress on the lumbar spine.

263. The answer is D.

In a Romberg test, a patient is asked to maintain an erect stance with the eyes open. If this portion of the test is performed satisfactorily, then the patient must maintain erect stance with the eyes closed. A loss of balance with the eyes closed suggests that the patient relies on visual input.

264. The answer is A.

Patients with Parkinson's disease usually ambulate with the trunk in flexion. Increased trunk flexion causes a festinating gait to be more pronounced. Therapy should strengthen extensor muscles while stretching the flexors. Slow rocking has been shown to decrease tone, and biofeedback can improve a gait with shorter step and stride length by placing of markers on the floor for the feet.

265. The answer is A.

The anterior cruciate ligament prevents excessive posterior roll of the femoral condyles during flexion of the femur at the knee joint.

266. The answer is C.

Postural reactions and motor milestone development occur in the same sequence as with normal infants, but the progression of an infant with Down's syndrome is slower.

267. The answer is C.

Standing positions have less of a base of support than sitting. In addition, standing on a foam block challenges the ankle's proprioceptive ability.

268. The answer is B.

Full-body immersion in a warm whirlpool is contraindicated in this scenario for two reasons. The blood vessels throughout the submerged portion of the body will dilate, causing a rapid change in blood pressure. This alteration in hemodynamic status may cause fainting. In addition, heat may not be able to dissipate from the body if the surrounding water is at a temperature higher than body temperature. This increases the risk for heat-related illnesses.

269. The answer is D.

Ultrasound dosages remain the same for phonophoresis as for regular ultrasound. This is true regardless of the medication used.

270. The answer is C.

Transverse (perpendicular to the scar) or circular massage assists in mobilization of scar tissue.

271. The answer is A.

After the first 2 years of life, the femurs rotate to a more neutral position, and the amount of anteversion decreases.

272. The answer is D.

Although vibration often elicits a muscle contraction, PTAs should first choose stimuli that are more likely to occur naturally.

273. The answer is A.

Bottle or breast feeding is rarely performed successfully before 34 weeks, gestational age. A sidelying position allows the infant to move the hands toward the mouth. The prone position encourages flexion. Full contact with the hand is more comforting to the infant.

274. The answer is A.

If the involved hand is fixed on a firm surface, the anterior deltoid and pectoralis major function to adduct the humerus. Adduction of the proximal humerus in this position causes slight medial movement of the distal humerus. This combination of movements locks the elbow in extension. A C6 quadriplegic does not have adequate triceps muscles because they are innervated by C7.

275. The answer is C.

This position, which limits inversion, plantarflexion, and adduction, is the most common position for ankle sprains.

276. The answer is B.

The thoracic pads should be on the inferior/lateral chest wall.

277. The answer is C.

The classification is no activity = 0; slight contraction = 1+; normal response = 2+; exaggerated response = 3+; severely exaggerated = 4+.

278. The answer is C.

A tissue stretch end-feel is also felt with ankle dorsiflexion. An example of a bone-to-bone end-feel is with knee or elbow extension. Knee flexion is an example of soft tissue approximation. In an empty end-feel, a patient stops the movement because of pain.

279. The answer is A.

Avoiding the interossei helps to inhibit tone. Direct pressure to any hand musculature may increase tone. Hyperextension of the MCP joints may also cause an increase in tone.

280. The answer is A.

With the safety button, the patient can stop the traction at any point. If any of the other choices are set incorrectly, the patient can stop the machine before damage is done.

281. The answer is B.

Volumetrics are appropriate for the distal portion of the extremities, such as the hand and foot. Submerging the entire extremity is not only time consuming, but it may not be accurate enough to detect small changes in girth in proximal joints. Subjective observation is not as accurate as objective girth measurements.

282. The answer is C.

Functional tests are often used to measure a patient's level of function as it relates to normal life.

283. The answer is B.

The biceps is tested with the forearm in supination, and the brachioradialis is tested with the forearm midway between pronation and supination.

284. The answer is B.

Interferential current stimulators are high-frequency units that use two separate AC channels and usually four electrodes.

285. The answer is A.

Interferential current stimulators and transcutaneous electrical nerve stimulation units are used for pain control, and DC is used to promote wound healing. Some sources advocate pulsed, rhythmic AC stimulation to decrease edema. Muscle strengthening protocols usually involve one channel with a frequency between 50 and 80 pulses per second.

286. The answer is A.

Isometric control develops before isotonic control.

287. The answer is C.

A macerated wound is excessively moist and requires a dressing to decrease the moisture to an acceptable level. A wound that is hardened would be described as indurated and would require a moist dressing. An antiobiotic dressing is used to prevent or reduce infection. A wound that is covered with eschar is often treated with an enzymatic debrider.

288. The answer is C.

A prolonged stretch assists in decreasing tone.

289. The answer is D.

Movements that stress the posterolateral hip joint capsule should be avoided. Sources vary on the exact amount of flexion that should be avoided. Passive hip abduction should be maintained after surgery with a wedge.

290. The answer is D.

The prone and sidelying positions would encourage flexion of the extremities with this patient. In this population, prone positioning allows more efficient cardiovascular function.

291. The answer is A.

Exercise should be terminated if oxygen saturation falls below 88%.

292. The answer is A.

Hydrostatic (underwater) weighing involves comparing body weight in and out of water. Electrical impedance involves the principle that lean tissues have a greater electrolyte content than fat. Impedance measurements have a high margin of error. Anthropometric (skinfold) measurements also have a high margin of error, especially when made by unskilled individuals.

293. The answer is D.

A physical therapist or PTA cannot reveal information on another patient because it is a breach in confidentiality, regardless of whether or not the other person is a relative.

294. The answer is A.

Because of poor balance, geriatric patients should increase the treadmill grade rather than the speed. Use of machines allows better posture and low intensities and limits the exercise within the patient's safe ROM.

295. The answer is B.

A patient should always exhale during the exertion phase of an exercise such as abdominal crunches. Not doing so can cause an increase in blood pressure and an increase in pressure in the thoracic cage.

296. The answer is B.

According to the American Heart Association, an infant is considered to be younger than 1 year of age and should be assessed at the brachial artery for signs of circulation. A child is considered to be 1 to 8 years old and should be assessed at the carotid artery for signs of circulation. An adult is considered to be older than 8 years old and should also be assessed at the carotid artery.

297. The answer is D.

Herpes zoster involves a particular dorsal root and its ganglia. TENS unit electrodes should be placed over the involved dermatome (L5 in this case).

298. The answer is B.

The muscles of mastication are buccinator, lateral pterygoid, masseter, medial pterygoid, and temporalis. The platysma is considered to be a muscle of facial expression.

299. The answer is D.

All of the above are important skills for a patient with a hip disarticulation prosthesis to master, but posterior pelvic tilt should be mastered first to advance the prosthesis.

300. The answer is B.

Blisters should be allowed to subside naturally. Gel inserts lose their shape if not left in the prosthesis overnight. The prosthesis should be propped up in a corner or laid on the floor to prevent it from falling and cracking.

301. The answer is A.

If a muscle is positioned across two joints such that it is in its maximum shortened position, the muscle is at a mechanical disadvantage and will not be able to generate a strong contraction. This is referred to as active insufficiency. If a muscle is stretched across two joints such that it is in its most lengthened position, it is also at a mechanical disadvantage. This is referred to as passive insufficiency.

302. The answer is C.

This test assesses the strength of the latissimus dorsi. One of the functions of the latissimus is to push up from a sitting position. This test simulates that movement.

303. The answer is B.

The shrinker should be removed only for bathing. Because the surgical scars are healed, the stump can be immersed in water.

304. The answer is B.

The flexor digitorum profundus has four tendons, each attaching to the distal phalanx. If the three mentioned in the question are restricted, flexion at the distal interphalangeal joint in the normal hand would not be possible.

305. The answer is B.

In closed-chain activity, the femur medially rotates on the tibia. In open-chain activity, the tibia laterally rotates on the femur.

306. The answer is A.

The popliteus, biceps femoris, and iliotibial band offer active restraint for the lateral side of the knee joint. The gastrocnemius assists in active restraint of the posterior side of the knee joint.

307. The answer is D.

Acetic acid is sometimes used in attempts to dissolve a calcium deposit and is driven by the negative pole. Dexamethasone is an antiinflammatory agent driven by the negative pole. Magnesium sulfate is used to decrease muscle spasms and is driven by the positive pole. Hydrocortisone is also used to treat inflammation and is driven by the positive pole.

308. The answer is C.

The heart receives nerve impulses that travel through the sinoatrial node to the ventricles by way of the atrioventricular node, bundle branches, and Purkinje fibers.

309. The answer is A.

Although this rate is high, tachycardia is used to describe a rate greater than 100 bpm. Normal range is 60 to 100 bpm. Any rate below 60 bpm is described as bradycardia.

310. The answer is C.

Increasing motor ability is not independent of motor learning. A PTA must facilitate motor learning with proper sensory cues and by promoting appropriate motor activity. Answer D is true because infants begin with spontaneous movement, which later develops into more deliberate movement. Answer A is true because reflex movement can be used to develop more deliberate movement.

311. The answer is B.

Frothy sputum is thin and white or has a slight pink color. This type of sputum is commonly present with pulmonary edema. Purulent sputum resembles pus, with a yellow or green color. Mucopurulent sputum is yellow to light green in color. Rusty sputum is a rust-colored sputum often associated with pneumonia.

312. The answer is C.

Mucoid sputum is clear or white and is not usually associated with infection. Thick sputum is referred to as tenacious. Foul-smelling sputum is called fetid and is often associated with infection.

313. The answer is D.

The PTA does not need to wear a gown, gloves, or a mask. These precautions are necessary only if there is a chance that the assistant or his clothing can become contaminated with blood, serum, or feces.

314. The answer is A.

The average adult wheelchair width is 26 inches, but the opening should be at least 32 inches to allow for hand clearance. A wheelchair ramp should be built with a 1:12 slope. The toilet seat needs to be between 17 and 19 inches in height.

315. The answer is B.

The range considered "warm" for water settings in a whirlpool is between 35.5°C and 36.5°C, which is approximately 96°F to 98°F. The formula for converting Celsius to Fahrenheit is $F = (C \times 9/5) + 32$.

316. The answer is D.

This patient has a lesion at the level of C7.

317. The answer is A.

Adrenocorticotropic hormone, thyroid-stimulating hormone, growth hormone, follicle-stimulating hormone, and luteinizing hormone are all produced by the anterior pituitary gland. Insulin and glucagon are produced in the pancreas. Epinephrine and norepinephrine are produced in the adrenal medulla. Cortisol, androgens, and aldosterone are produced by the adrenal cortex.

318. The answer is D.

The radial side is the lateral side of the forearm, which is innervated by the musculocutaneous nerve. The lateral antebrachial cutaneous nerve is a continuation of the musculocutaneous nerve.

319. The answer is A.

Flexion and extension of the thumb are performed in a plane parallel to the palm of the hand. Abduction and adduction are performed in a plane perpendicular to the palm of the hand.

320. The answer is D.

This type of movement, known as athetosis, can also involve the feet, proximal parts of the extremities, and face. Chorea is rapid movements of the hands, wrist, or face. Ballism is a forceful and uncontrollable throwing of the extremities outward. Lead-pipe rigidity is increasing resistance of an extremity to passive ranging. All of the above can result from damage to the basal ganglia.

321. The answer is D.

This type of stimulation is usually not well tolerated by patients with acute conditions. Acute conditions are usually treated by TENS with a high frequency, and chronic conditions can be treated with a low frequency (if tolerated by the patient). Treatments providing a noxious stimulus usually have a longer-lasting effect.

322. The answer is B.

Pulmonary edema is primarily a result of left-sided heart failure.

323. The answer is D.

This is an example of Russian stimulation.

324. The answer is B.

These signs are characteristic of an arterial insufficiency ulcer. Patients with venous ulcers often present with the following symptoms: no pain around the wound, no gangrene, location typically on the medial ankle, pigmented skin around the ulcer, and significant edema. A trophic ulcer (also known as a pressure or decubitus ulcer) presents with decreased sensation, callused skin, no pain, and is located over bony prominences.

325. The answer is D.

After the cross-bridge attaches to the thin filament (or actin), it moves, causing the thin filament to move. After the cross-bridge is broken, it moves into position to reattach to a thin filament (or actin) to repeat the cycle.

326. The answer is D.

Answer A increases strength of the scalenes and sternocleidomastoid. Answer B strengthens the latissimus dorsi. Answer C increases the strength of the upper trapezius. All of these are accessory inspiratory muscles. Answer D strengthens the abdominals, which are muscles of forceful expiration.

327. The answer is A.

Fine motor control tasks require smaller pieces of material than large motor tasks. Gross motor skill activities also require larger movements, using larger muscle groups (thus requiring higher energy expenditure), than fine motor tasks. Fine motor activities also require a higher degree of accuracy.

328. The answer is D.

The incentive spirometer provides visual feedback of maximal inspiratory efforts. The PTA is qualified to answer the patient's question.

329. The answer is B.

Supine positioning after the first trimester is associated with decreased cardiac output.

330. The answer is B.

During periods of acute exacerbation, patients with multiple sclerosis should avoid any exertion.

331. The answer is C.

Residual volume, the amount of air left in the lungs after a forceful expiration, increases with age.

332. The answer is B.

While in place, positioning equipment limits a child's response to the environment.

333. The answer is B.

The external abdominal oblique flexes, ipsilaterally side bends, and contralaterally rotates the trunk.

334. The answer is B.

This is a description of a dystrophic gait pattern, also called penguin gait. Patients with muscular dystrophy commonly demonstrate this gait pattern. A gluteus maximus gait presents with the patient leaning the trunk back while striking the heel on the involved side (or lurching). An arthrogenic gait pattern presents with the patient circumducting and elevating the hip on the involved side. This pattern is present with severe stiffness or a fused joint in the involved lower extremity. An antalgic gait pattern is exhibited when a person has pain with weight bearing on the involved lower extremity.

335. The answer is D.

PNF diagonals are named according to the movement that will take place. The starting position is at a point that allows the maximum amount of movement. D1 flexion moves the hip into external rotation, flexion, and adduction. The knee may be in a flexed or extended position while the ankle is moving into inversion and dorsiflexion.

336. The answer is C.

Carpal tunnel syndrome often results from repetitive overuse of the hand. Typical signs and symptoms include pain, numbness, or tingling along the median nerve distribution of the hand; weak pinch strength; atrophy of the thenar muscles; and Tinel's sign.

337. The answer is C.

Activation of the sympathetic nervous system causes dilatation of the pupils, increased heart rate, increased blood pressure, activation of muscles, decreased peristalsis, and increased respiration.

338. The answer is B.

This patient is likely to experience a decrease in the number of red blood cells. All of the other statements are correct. Fibrinogen decreases initially but then increases throughout recovery.

339. The answer is D.

This answer lists the stages of control in the correct order.

340. The answer is B.

The pattern described in the question—a gradual increase in the rate and depth of respirations followed by periods of absent breathing—is known as Cheyne-Stokes breathing. Small breaths followed by inconsistent periods of absent breathing are known as a Biot's breathing pattern. Deep, gasping breaths are known as a Kussmaul's breathing pattern. Awakening during the night because of periods of absent breathing is known as paroxysmal nocturnal dyspnea.

341. The answer is A.

The talipes equinovarus foot is in the position of pes cavus, forefoot adduction, and rear foot varus.

342. The answer is D.

Apneusis can be described as an inspiratory cramp. Orthopnea is difficulty with breathing in a lying postion. Eupnea is normal breathing. Apnea is the absence of breathing.

343. The answer is D.

Patients with mild pes planus present with 4° to 6° of hind foot valgus and 4° to 6° of forefoot varus. The foot with moderate pes planus has 6° to 10° of hind foot valgus and 6° to 10° of forefoot varus.

344. The answer is C.

A person is usually diagnosed with type I diabetes at age 25 years or younger. A person is usually age 40 years or older when diagnosed with type II diabetes. Ketoacidosis is a symptom of type I diabetes. Metabolism of free fatty acids in the liver causes this condition, which is an excess of ketones. A type II diabetic may be able to control his or her condition with diet only (depending on the severity of the condition), but a type I diabetic needs insulin.

345. The answer is D.

The Landau reaction (onset at 4 months, integrated at 24 months) is assessed by supporting the patient in prone position and passively or actively extending the neck. A positive response is extension of the spine and lower extremities. The Moro reflex is tested by lowering an infant suddenly from a sitting position. A positive response is crying with sudden extension and abduction of the upper extremities, followed by adduction of the upper extremities across the chest (an infant should have this response at up to 6 months of age). Labyrinthine head righting is tested by holding a child upright and tilting the body slightly forward, back, and side to side. The infant should be able to hold the head vertical despite the body movement. The symmetric tonic neck response (onset at 4–6 months; integrated at 8–12 months) is exhibited when the infant displays upper extremity extension and lower extremity flexion with passive cervical extension. Sources vary significantly in regard to the age at which these responses should be present and when they are integrated.

346. The answer is D.

This is an example of an associated reaction, which presents from birth to age 3 months and is integrated at age 9 years. The Landau reaction (onset at 4 months; integrated at 24 months) is assessed by supporting the patient in prone position and passively or actively extending the neck. A positive response is extension of the spine and lower extremities. The startle reflex is positive if an infant is startled by a loud or sudden noise. This response should be present at birth and persists throughout life. The Moro reflex is tested by lowering an infant suddenly from a sitting position. A positive response is crying with sudden extension and abduction of the upper extremities, followed by adduction of the upper extremities across the chest (an infant should have this response up to age 6 months). Sources vary significantly in regard to the age at which these responses should be present and when they are integrated.

347. The answer is A.

The splenius cervicis muscles function to extend, ipsilaterally rotate, and ipsilaterally side bend the cervical spine.

348. The answer is D.

All of the listed muscles participate in mandibular elevation with the exception of the lateral pterygoid muscle. The lateral pterygoid muscle and the suprahyoid muscles participate in mandibular depression.

349. The answer is D.

When a patient with Parkinson's disease has been using levodopa for an extended period, he or she may develop resistance to the medication. Sometimes a break from the drug for 7 to 10 days may enhance its effectiveness.

350. The answer is B.

A flexible pes planus foot is defined as a decreased medial longitudinal arch in weight bearing but normal medial longitudinal arch in non–weight bearing.

351. The answer is B.

A tennis elbow band is believed to align the tendons in a more parallel position, versus a bowed position without the band, which decreases the amount of stretch on the tendons.

352. The answer is B.

Passive extension is the most important motion to gain after an anterior cruciate ligament reconstruction, regardless of the graft type. Active extension can be achieved after passive extension is full (or equal bilaterally).

353. The answer is D.

The elbow joint is in a loose packed position when the elbow is between 70° and 90° of flexion.

354. The answer is B.

A patient with a diagnosis of spinal stenosis will experience an exacerbation of symptoms with lumbar extension exercises. Lumbar flexion exercises are indicated.

355. The answer is A.

AIDS is transmitted by blood or bodily fluids. Masks are usually used with airborne precautions. Handwashing should be done between all wound care patients. Gloves are also indicated with all open wounds. Gowns may not be a necessity but should be used if there is a chance of soiling the clothing with infected fluids.

356. The answer is B.

Iontophoresis uses direct current to drive medication through the skin by repelling ions. For example, if a medication is positively charged, it can be driven by the anode (the positive electrode); if a medication is negatively charged, it can be driven by the cathode (the negative electrode).

357. The answer is D.

This patient is most likely experiencing lumbar radiculopathy. Although McKenzie extension exercises are appropriate, the supervising therapist must be informed because these exercises were not part of the original plan of care.

358. The answer is C.

This is a description of the petrissage technique. Effleurage is stroking of the skin. Friction massages are used to mobilize scar tissue. Tapotement is tapping of the skin.

359. The answer is B.

There is minimal ligament damage with a grade 1 sprain of the AC joint. Usually there is no palpable disruption in the AC joint. A grade 3 injury involves a complete tear of the acromioclavicular and coracoacromial ligaments.

360. The answer is C.

Patients with chronic obstructive airway disease are often given this set of instructions, which is known as the method of pursed-lips breathing. This method helps patients regain control of their breathing rate and increase tidal volume and amount of oxygen absorbed.

361. The answer is D.

Men with high complete lesions are likely to be able to have reflexogenic erections, and men with lower complete lesions are likely to have the capability to have reflexogenic or psychogenic erections. Men with incomplete lesions are likely to retain erectile capability much more than men with complete lesions. In addition, men with complete lesions are less likely to have the ability to ejaculate than men with incomplete lesions.

362. The answer is D.

To perform a lift correctly, the pelvis should be anteriorly rotated before lifting objects from the floor.

363. The answer is A.

Patients with decerebrate rigidity are positioned with all extremities extended and the wrist and fingers flexed. Patients with decorticate posturing are positioned with the upper extremities flexed, the lower extremities hyperextended, and the fingers tightly flexed.

364. The answer is A.

The patient is using palmar prehension in this scenario. Palmar prehension is holding an object between the thumb pad and the middle and index finger. Fingertip prehension is used when a person picks up an object between the thumb pad and either the index or middle finger (not both at the same time, as with palmar prehension). In lateral prehension, the thumb pad is in contact with the lateral side of the index finger proximal to the distal interphalangeal joint. In a hook grasp, the fingers are flexed as if carrying a bucket by the handle. The thumb does not provide much active movement when the hook grasp is used.

365. The answer is C.

The crutches are held by the grips with the hand on the uninvolved side to transfer from sit to stand.

366. The answer is A.

A patient of this age usually can begin using crutches instead of a standard walker. If the patient has no cognitive deficits and was independent in ambulation without an assistive device before surgery, she then most likely will have the balance and coordination necessary to ambulate with crutches. A three-point gait pattern is necessary because of the current partial weight-bearing status. A swing-to pattern also can be used, but a three-point pattern assists more quickly in returning to a more normal gait pattern.

367. The answer is B.

Pressure on the left temporal bone just anterior to the ear helps to occlude blood flow from the temporal artery.

368. The answer is A.

A ground fault interruption circuit protects the patient from a potentially life-threatening situation. The other choices are valid concerns, but A is the most important one.

369. The answer is A.

Because the interossei cross the MP joints and PIP joints, the PIP joints should be flexed with the MP joints in flexion and extension.

370. The answer is D.

The first sound heard corresponds with closing of the mitral and tricuspid valves. The second sound corresponds to closing of the aortic and pulmonic valves. Therefore, the first sound indicates the onset of ventricular systole, and the second sound indicates the onset of ventricular diastole.

371. The answer is D.

This sequence assists in propelling the center of gravity forward to maintain balance after a backward sway.

372. The answer is C.

Answer C is incorrect. Heat decreases spasm by causing the vessels to dilate, which brings more blood (containing oxygen) to the area. Cold decreases spasm by decreasing sensitivity of the muscle spindles.

373. The answer is A.

The patella moves superiorly during knee extension and inferiorly during flexion. The tibia should be mobilized according to the concave–convex rule.

374. The answer is A.

A Bankhart lesion occurs when the anterior rim of the glenoid labrum is pulled away from the glenoid fossa during an anterior dislocation of the shoulder.

375. The answer is B.

Answer B is correct because the patient has to achieve passive knee extension before she can gain full active knee extension. Full active knee extension and full flexion are important and should be a major focus of the patient's session, but the question asks for the most serious deficit. Ambulating with a lesser assistive device should be the focus at a later time because the patient's gait is still severely antalgic and obvious instability is still present. Usually a patient is advanced to a lesser assistive device when he or she can ambulate without large gait deviations with the current assistive device.

376. The answer is B.

This is an example of a bipolar configuration. Another form of bipolar configuration is to have two electrodes of equal size, each from a different lead wire. In a monopolar configuration, one smaller electrode is placed over the intended site and a larger electrode is placed some distance away. The stimulation is perceived by the patient, in this case, only under the smaller electrode. In a quadripolar configuration, two electrodes coming from two different lead wires are placed over the intended area.

377. The answer is C.

Placing a plug-in unit close to water pipes is a potential hazard because it offers another possible ground pathway to the patient. Never use an extension cord or an adaptor with a plug-in unit. If the adaptor or cord does not have a ground prong, it may cause shock to the patient through a leaking current. If the machine intensity is adjusted during the off portion of the cycle, the stimulation may be too high for the patient when the on cycle returns.

378. The answer is D.

Flexion and abduction beyond 90° causes further impingement of the rotator cuff and usually increases the patient's subjective complaints of pain. After pain has subsided, exercise above 90° can usually begin within tolerable pain limits.

379. The answer is C.

The electromyogram (EMG) does not record torque. Instead, it assists by showing a linear relationship between the EMG and the force produced by the muscle during an isometric contraction.

380. The answer is D.

In order to perform the exercise correctly, the poundage should be decreased. Also moving the weight proximally would decrease the moment arm from the hip and therefore decrease the force required to accomplish a correct straight leg raise.

381. The answer is D.

Answer A is contraindicated because the electromagnetic field produced by use of short-wave diathermy or microwave diathermy may alter the settings of a pacemaker. Answer B is contraindicated because the metal heats quickly and may cause the surrounding tissue to heat excessively, potentially causing a burn. Answer C is contraindicated because heating causes vasodilation, making a hemorrhage more likely. Answer D is the correct choice because pulsed short-wave diathermy can be used on patients with acute or chronic conditions. With most pulsed short-wave treatments, there is no measurable temperature increase in the tissues.

382. The answer is B.

The dorsalis pedis artery is a branch of the anterior tibial artery. The anterior tibial artery can be compressed by edema in the anterior compartment.

383. The answer is B.

Closed-chain exercises are performed when the distal segment of the extremity is bearing weight or fixed. In open-chain activities, the distal segment is free to move.

384. The answer is B.

Sedentary patients' cardiovascular responses increase faster than trained patients' responses if the workloads are equal.

385. The answer is D.

The geriatric population usually has a decreased body temperature caused by poor diet, decreased cardiovascular status, and decreased metabolic rates.

386. The answer is C.

Fully elevating the leg rests of the patient's chair increases hip flexion. The already tight hamstrings (secondary to contracture) would tilt the pelvis posterior. This maneuver would increase weight on the ischial tuberosity, risking a decubitus ulcer. Choice D is correct because sliding board transfers can lead to abrasions. Choices A and B are also correct measures to decrease the chance of developing ulcers.

387. The answer is A.

Patients with ideomotor apraxia can often identify objects but cannot use them correctly on command. Such patients often can perform the activity spontaneously. Patients with ideational apraxia often cannot identify objects or use them. Both situations call for short one-step commands.

388. The answer is D.

The Romberg test is a type of equilibrium test. Whereas equilibrium tests are usually conducted with the patient in a standing position, nonequilibrium tests are performed with the patient in the supine position.

389. The answer is C.

Trigger points are often treated with soft tissue massage. Other techniques include strain/counterstrain, myofascial release, and muscle energy techniques.

390. The answer is B.

Flexor withdrawal is tested by the introduction of a painful stimulus to the sole of the foot. The knee and hip flex to avoid the stimulus. In proprioceptive placing, the dorsum of the infant's foot touches the edge of a table. The infant then brings the foot to the tabletop. The spontaneous stepping reflex is displayed when the infant is supported with the feet lightly touching a firm surface. The infant will make stepping motions as he or she is moved forward.

391. The answer is C.

A child with excessive flexion of the toes during weight bearing will have difficulty ambulating.

392. The answer is A.

Back blows should be followed by chest thrusts with complete airway obstruction when cardiopulmonary resuscitation is performed on an infant. The PTA should then check for a foreign body in the airway. A blind finger sweep of the throat should not be performed on infants.

393. The answer is D.

The assistant should contact the physical therapist. The physical therapist can then make the determination on whether the physician should be contacted.

394. The answer is C.

Answer C provides correct instructions. The patient is often instructed to begin this technique in the supine position and progress to the sitting position. This technique should be practiced for approximately 5 minutes several times per day.

395. The answer is B.

Answer A is true because near-infrared lamps can penetrate up to 10 mm compared with 2 mm with far-infrared lamps. Answer B is a false statement because infrared lamps can heat only one side of an extremity at a time. Answers C and D are true statements because the intensity of the infrared lamp can be changed by altering the angle of the beam with the treated part or the distance between the body part and the lamp.

396. The answer is C.

The right shoulder and thorax begin to move forward at heel strike (i.e., initial contact).

397. The answer is D.

The fingers can be bound in paraffin wax as well as in fluidotherapy. When using this technique, the hand remains stationary throughout the heating process, which is necessary for paraffin to be most effective (when using the standard method of dipping the hand and wrapping with plastic wrap and a towel).

398. The answer is B.

Although the change may be minimal, increasing the maximal pressure to 60 mm Hg is the most likely choice to have a positive affect on edema reduction. The BP, however, should not exceed the diastolic BP of the patient. Answer A is not the right choice because placing the extremity in a dependent position causes the pump to work against gravity. Answer C is incorrect because decreasing the on time means that the extremity receives compression for a shorter period. Answer D is incorrect because greater pressure distally is more likely to move fluid than equal pressure throughout the sleeve.

399. The answer is D.

Because the physician is asking for an opinion about this patient's diagnosis, the supervising therapist should speak directly to the physician. The determination of a rotator cuff tear requires special testing, usually performed during the evaluation.

400. The answer is C.

Raynaud's phenomenon is a vasospastic disorder of the vessels of the distal parts of the extremities. Patients with Raynaud's phenomenon do not respond well to cold treatment. Choice B is incorrect because it is believed that moist heat may encourage more rapid growth of cancer. Choice D is incorrect because prolonged use of steroids may cause the capillaries to lose their integrity, which compromises the body's ability to dissipate heat. Choice A is incorrect because moist heat may encourage hemorrhaging in patients with hemophilia by causing vasodilation.

BIBLIOGRAPHY

1. Agur AMR: Grant's Atlas of Anatomy, 9th ed. Baltimore, Williams & Wilkins, 1991.

2. Brooks DS: Program Design for Personal Trainers: Bridging Theory into Application. Champaign, IL, Human Kinetics, 1978.

3. Charness A, Schneider FJ: Stroke/Head Injury: A Guide to Functional Outcomes in Physical Therapy Management. Gaithersburg, MD, Aspen Publishers, 1986.

4. Ciccone CD: Pharmacology in Rehabilitation. Philadelphia, F.A. Davis, 1996.

5. Clark PN, Allen AS: Occupational Therapy for Children. St Louis, MO, CV Mosby, 1985.

6. Connolly BH, Montgomery PC: Therapeutic Exercise in Developmental Disabilities, 2nd ed. Hixson, TN, Chattanooga Group, 1993.

7. Elston RC, Johnson WE: Essentials of Biostatistics, 2nd ed. Philadelphia, F.A. Davis, 1994.

8. Hayes KW: Manual for Physical Agents 5th ed. Norwalk CT, Appleton & Lange, 1999.

9. Hecox B, Wiesberg J, Mehreteab T: Physical Agents: A Comprehensive Text for Physical Therapists. Norwalk, CT, Appleton and Lange, 1994.

10. Hillegass EA, Sadowsky HS: Essentials of Cardiopulmonary Physical Therapy. Philadelphia, W.B. Saunders, 1994.

11. Hoppenfeld S: Physical Examination of the Spine and Extremities. Norwalk, CT, Appleton & Lange, 1976.

12. Jenkins DB: Hollinshead's Functional Anatomy of the Limbs and Back, 6th ed. Philadelphia, W.B. Saunders, 1991.

13. Karacoloff LA, Hammersley CS, Schneider FJ: Lower Extremity Amputation, 2nd ed. Gaithersburg, MD, Aspen Publishers, 1992.

14. Kenney WL, Humphrey RH, Bryant CX: ASCM's Guidelines for Exercise Testing and Prescription, 5th ed. Baltimore, Williams & Wilkins, 1995.

15. Kettenbach G: Writing SOAP Notes, 2nd ed. Philadelphia, F.A. Davis, 1995.

16. Kisner C, Colby LA: Therapeutic Exercise: Foundations and Techniques. 4th ed. Philadelphia, F.A. Davis, 2002.

17. Liebler JG, Levine RE, Rothman J: Management Principles for Health Professionals, 2nd ed. Gaithersburg, MD, Aspen Publishers, 1992.

18. Lippert L: Clinical Kinesiology for Physical Therapist Assistants, 3rd ed. Philadelphia, F.A. Davis, 2000.

19. Magee DJ: Orthopedic Physical Assessment, 3rd ed. Philadelphia, W.B. Saunders, 1997.

20. Marieb E: Human Anatomy and Physiology. Redwood City, CA, Benjamin/Cummings, 1992.

21. Minor MA, Minor SD: Patient Care Skills, 3rd ed. Norwalk, CT, Appleton & Lange, 1995.

22. Minor MA, Minor SD: Patient Care Skills, 4th ed. Norwalk, CT, Appleton & Lange, 1998.

23. Michlovitz SL: Thermal Agents in Rehabilitation, 2nd ed. Philadelphia, F.A. Davis, 1990.

24. Michlovitz SL: Thermal Agents in Rehabilitation, 3rd ed. Philadelphia, F.A. Davis, 1996.

25. Netter FH: Atlas of Human Anatomy. Summit, NJ, Ciba-Geigy Corporation, 1989.

26. Noback CR, Stominger NL, Demarest RJ: The Human Nervous System, 4th ed. Philadelphia, Lea & Febiger, 1991.

27. Norkin CC, Levangie PK: Joint Structure and Function, 3rd ed. Philadelphia, F.A. Davis, 2001.

28. Norkin CC, White DJ: Measurement of Joint Motion, 3rd ed. Philadelphia, F.A. Davis, 2003.

29. Novak TJ, Handford AG: Essentials of Pathophysiology. Dubuque, IA, William C. Brown, 1994.

30. Montgomery PC, Connolly BH: Motor Control and Physical Therapy, 2nd ed. Hixson, TN, Chattanooga Group, 1995.

31. O'Sullivan SB, Schmitz TJ: Physical Rehabilitation Assessment and Treatment, 4th ed. Philadelphia, F.A. Davis, 2001.

32. Pedretti LW: Occupational Therapy: Practice Skills for Physical Dysfunction, 4th ed. St. Louis, Mosby, 1996.

33. Rancho Los Amigos Medical Center: Observational Gait Analysis. Rancho Los Amigos Medical Center, Downy, CA, 1993.

34. Richardson JK, Iglarsh ZA: Clinical Orthopaedic Physical Therapy, Philadelphia, W.B. Saunders, 1994.

35. Robinson AJ, Synder-Mackler L: Clinical Electrophysiology, 2nd ed. Baltimore, Williams & Wilkins, 1995.

36. Rothstein JM, Roy SH, Wolf SL: The Rehabilitation Specialist Handbook, 2nd ed. Philadelphia, F.A. Davis, 1998.

37. Scully RM, Barnes MR: Physical Therapy. Philadelphia, J.B. Lippincott, 1989.

38. Shankman, G: Fundamental Orthopedic Management for the Physical Therapist Assistant. St. Louis, MO, Mosby, 1997.

39. Starkey C: Therapeutic Modalities for Athletic Trainers, 2nd ed. Philadelphia, F.A. Davis, 1998.

40. Sullivan PE, Markos PD: Clinical Decision Making in Therapeutic Exercise. Norwalk, CT, Appleton & Lange, 1995.

41. Summers MF: Spinal Cord Injury. Norwalk, CT, Appleton & Lange, 1992.

42. Tamparo C, Lewis M: Diseases of the Human Body, 3rd ed. Philadelphia, F.A. Davis, 1995.

43. Thomas CL: Taber's Cyclopedic Medical Dictionary, 19th ed. Philadelphia, F.A. Davis, 2001.

44. Tortora G, Grabowski S: Principles of Anatomy and Physiology, 7th ed. New York, Harper Collins, 1993.

45. Vander AJ, Sherman JH, Luciano DS: Human Physiology: The Mechansim of Body Function, New York, McGraw–Hill, 1994.

46. Williams SJ, Torrens PR: Introduction to Health Sciences, 4th ed. Albany NY, Delmar Publishers, 1993.